MAKE EVERY
SHOT COUNT

MAKE EVERY SHOT COUNT

How Basketball Taught a Point Guard to Be a Surgeon

BRUCE ROSENFELD, MD

Make Every Shot Count: How Basketball Taught a
Point Guard to Be a Surgeon, Revised Edition

Copyright © 2011, 2020 Bruce Rosenfeld.
All rights reserved.

Cover and book design by Sean Ford

ISBN 978-1-7337516-5-0

Printed in the United States of America

For Lisa and Ellen

Author's Note

All the stories here are true. However, to protect the confidentiality of patients, colleagues, and instructors in the medical portion of this book, I have changed the names. In addition, I have also had to alter minor identifying details in certain instances for the same reason.

MAKE EVERY
SHOT COUNT

Chapter One:

THE FIGHT

These guys were big. At least they seemed like giants compared to every other kid in our neighborhood. It was a special day; we had persuaded the two titans in our group to compete head-to-head in a boxing match. Promoted as a fight to the death, or at least until someone was bloodied beyond recognition, we hoped the contest would at least go until one of the kids was knocked out and couldn't get up, just like we'd seen in the pro fights on television. This would be an epic battle, and we couldn't control our excitement.

Despite being in fourth grade, our heroes and classmates Jimmy and Eppy were known for their size and strength at a time when those attributes brought you tremendous status and popularity. These guys were the first to be picked for any team, no matter the sport. They earned it; they were incredible athletes at a young age. Yet this distinction also carried great responsibility as the two felt pressured to produce the most points, hit the ball the farthest, and do whatever was necessary to win. I was small for my age and would have given almost anything to be their size.

The fight became possible only after one of the kids received boxing gloves for his birthday. We set the time, date, and location—Jimmy's backyard—well in advance. One of us then came up with the idea that we now needed to sell tickets. So we set the price at twenty-five cents each, figuring it was a bargain. But before the match could happen, we needed to set up a boxing ring. From there we got creative collecting fallen branches, sawed them off as needed, and hammered the straightest and most solid ones into the ground connecting them with household string to outline the area. Our construction was completed well before the big day, and despite the shoddy workmanship, we liked what we saw.

Kids raided their moms' pocketbooks to cover the cost, and the tickets sold quickly. No one wanted to miss this event. For days leading up to the fight, the trash-talking and predictions were nonstop. As promoters, we saw cash rolling in, yet if we'd been true entrepreneurs, we would have organized betting as well. That, however, was way beyond our level of sophistication.

It was a beautiful fall Saturday, and all of us, and especially the two fighters, were ready to go. Our guys stood tall, adorned with their best cotton gym shorts, Keds high-top sneakers, long white tube socks, and oversized bathrobes stolen from their fathers' closets. The backyard was packed with kids from up and down the block and some even farther away, all having yelled as they ran out the door that they were going out to play, never letting on to the significance of the day. Too excited for the big event, no one had been able to sleep the night before.

The match began as both fighters nodded at each other, dancing in their corners while working the crowd and acknowledging last-minute instructions from their trainers. As with all fights, a referee was required. One kid reluctantly assumed the role, explaining the rules loudly over the energized crowd. The two fighters stared each other down, assessing who would flinch first. We had all learned early that if you could identify fear in your opponent's eyes, you had already won. That lesson was carried on by most of us for years to come.

As the promoters of this event, we thought we had attended to every detail. The fighters had shorts, gloves, and robes, but we didn't notice they had no headgear, no mouthguards, and no training. Certainly no one had any idea how this was going to turn out. The two went back to their corners and the crowd began screaming, its pitch growing increasingly higher. The gloves were tightly laced, and the robes were ready to come off. It was time!

As each fighter was introduced by our MC in the best booming voice he could muster without a microphone, the two began to strip down. At that moment, it became obvious something was wrong—the boxing gloves could not squeeze through the bathrobe sleeves no matter how hard we stretched or pulled. We looked silly trying to help and eventually, we unlaced the gloves and removed them. The robes were taken off, and the gloves were replaced and tied back up. Despite the embarrassment, this incident delayed the fight only a few minutes. Luckily the crowd was understanding as this was our first major event. At nine and ten years old, we weren't concerned about what other miscalculations we might have made. There were way too many to count.

With a loud clang (or more accurately, a clunk of a hammer on a metal garbage can top), the contest began. The two fighters charged into the center of the ring, their fists swinging and flailing in all directions without an ounce of technique. Now, don't get me wrong, these two guys knew how to fight. We all did. On a weekly if not daily basis, each of us typically was involved in some altercation that escalated to throwing punches. That was just how we settled most arguments at the time. You yelled and hurled insults, you fought, and then you were friends again. But there had never been any formal training. So at the start of the first round, our two fighters lunged at each other in pure survival mode. Although they hit each other with a flurry of hard punches to the face and head, each fighter tried to avoid being the first to get knocked out or beaten too badly.

I'm not sure exactly what took place next since it all happened so quickly. Jimmy's mom, obviously aware of the event since the entire neighborhood had been in her backyard before the opening moment, had been watching through her kitchen window. When she realized this fight could turn ugly fast, she frantically ran out the back door, kicked aside the boxing ring, and forcefully separated the fighters. In a powerful voice, she ordered all of us out of the yard and promised to call each of our parents. The disappointed crowd scattered in all directions, trying to hide their faces as they ran.

Sure, as its promoters we were upset at the outcome (or the lack thereof) of the fight. But now we had one last dilemma. We held all the ticket money, yet from our perspective, it wasn't our fault that the fight was canceled by circumstances beyond our control. We tried to argue the point with the crowd once we had reconvened, but they saw it very differently. With their tempers flaring, we knew we had only one option. And that option was to run. So we ran. Yes, indeed, we ran as far and as fast as we could, money in hand. We hid in the nearby woods for several hours, waiting until things blew over. We figured it had been a good decision.

Handling conflict was an art that had to be learned at an early age; sometimes you fought, and sometimes you ran. This situation called for us to run as the odds were too steep to take a stand. As the years went by, we all learned other techniques for handling disputes, but unfortunately for many of us, that took far too long.

The year was 1967 and the location was Metuchen, New Jersey. Tract houses were crammed onto tiny parcels of land, all part of a quickly constructed development thirty miles from New York City. With only two styles of houses available, we all knew the layout of our buddies' homes even before walking through the door. That made it pretty easy to find the kitchen, the bathroom, or the usually off-limits living room with plastic-encased furniture.

From a young age, I knew the names and grades of every kid in the neighborhood—crucial information when organizing a game. Most households had a dad, a stay-at-home mom, and three children close in age. There was never a shortage of kids around for whatever you needed.

By your fifth birthday, a typical day began with you proclaiming, "I'm going out to play!" as you slammed the door behind you and ran out to join your friends, never waiting for an answer. From that point on, you would hang out either on the street or in a backyard. The only rule was to be home for dinner or call to say where you were. Adults were never around when we organized our play, and the group spanned all ages. The younger kids idolized the older, listening intently as they recounted their middle school or high school drama. We didn't understand a lot about their experiences, and most of what we were exposed to would not be considered age-appropriate today. But we needed to hear everything for our own futures, and we asked a lot of questions. Television was only a minor influence on us, and there were no such things as computers, cell phones, or video games. It was up to us to create our entertainment.

Often, a group would walk up and down the street, gathering kids to come out and play. It was rare that any of our friends weren't allowed to tag along, since all our parents were eager to get us out of the house. Only one family in the neighborhood had a swimming pool, and if the weather was hot enough, we'd drop in on those kids to check their plans for the day, always wearing bathing suits and holding beach towels. This strategy was never effective, but that didn't stop us from trying—and trying often.

Our favorite activity was setting up and playing any kind of sport, depending on the weather and time of year, but it was usually baseball, basketball, or football. When wanting to be more creative, we'd organize a war game, choosing sides and making up rules that changed as the contest proceeded. This usually involved chasing each other around the neighborhood launching whatever we could find as ammunition— anything from snowballs to dirt bombs to rocks. If you were hit, the other team would earn points. These contests were fought over hours and sometimes even days. Or at least until one team surrendered, which almost never happened. More often, we'd just get bored or someone would get injured.

Whatever activity we dreamed up, winning was always the objective. We understood the importance of being the victor, and did everything we could to claim that title. You just never wanted to be on the losing side and without our understanding, that objective shaped our approach to life.

Chapter Two:

WHAT'S WRONG WITH THIS KID?

The grade-school experience in 1960s Metuchen was probably similar to the experience of any of the hundreds of suburban towns surrounding New York City. A bicycle was our standard mode of transportation, which allowed us not to rely on our parents for rides. This fostered our early independence. We all thought our town was pretty safe, and it was, more so than many that bordered us. In this part of New Jersey, you could drive for twenty minutes on the same busy road, mostly lined with strip malls and single businesses, and pass through a half dozen towns, each with its own reputation and characteristics. Some you might stop at with your folks to go into a store, while others you wanted to get through as quickly as possible with the windows and doors shut tightly.

In Metuchen, families tended to leave their front doors unlocked, although this never made any sense to me, since most of the families I knew had been robbed at least once. Kids would commonly walk alone, even at night without concern, yet being threatened by a group in a car was not that unusual. Due to the constant harassment of young people in this era, both provoked and unprovoked, none of us trusted the police and wouldn't consider involving them in any of our concerns. Our parents had grown up in a more innocent and trusting time and were naïve enough to believe that all was still the same. But the world had changed. Unlike today, there were no such things as play dates; we were simply expected to create our own diversion.

As emphasized, the most popular sports among all the neighborhood kids were baseball, basketball, and football. Both girls and boys of all ages played, and the hierarchy that eventually developed was based not on age or sex but on skill. It was acceptable to talk trash, but you had better be able to back it up on the court or the field or wherever the competition was being held. We also built and rode on homemade skateboards, set up obstacle courses, and had races of all kinds, constantly competing for supremacy in speed, agility, and strength. Whenever we had snowfall, the sleds came out for racing. We also had snowball fights and demonstrated our accuracy by pelting the windshields of passing cars, both scaring and angering their occupants. We usually ended up running from the drivers who jumped out of their cars to pummel the perpetrators. We knew they would never catch us, but the excitement was part of the challenge.

We made up hundreds of games. Some caught on and others didn't; what mattered most was how fast you could run or how far you could throw or spit or, for that matter, pee (one contest definitely restricted to the boys). No matter what we did, it was always about competition; that was how you garnered status in our world.

I finished elementary school in June 1969, and most of my memories from that time occurred outside the classroom. I rarely worked hard or was motivated in school, which didn't bother me at all. Once, on report-card day, my fourth-grade teacher asked me to speak with her at lunch. She told me I'd received straight A's and was the first student to earn this honor. It seemed like a big deal to her, but it didn't matter to me at all. It might have been the only time I had applied myself in elementary school, and I didn't do nearly as well in the grades before or after.

My dad was a successful physician in obstetrics and gynecology. Our lives were hectic, and my parents were busy, both professionally and socially. At this time, being a doctor was a calling rather than a career, and the time commitment was massive. It was not uncommon for me to go three or four days in a row without seeing my father, as he often delivered babies until late at night and left for the hospital again before I woke up in the morning. This was his life, and those were the expectations of a physician. I never questioned the hours or resented him for his obligation. On the contrary, I was proud to have a father who was a physician. My mother had her projects but was always available and kept the family organized and grounded. However, I had two other siblings, so her time had to be divided among all of us.

By the time I completed the fifth grade at Moss Elementary School, I was a fairly independent eleven-year-old and a decent athlete but with no focus on a specific sport. Yet for whatever reason, I was starting to feel as if I didn't fit in anywhere. I was distancing myself from others and getting into trouble at school. I didn't understand what was happening to me. My parents saw the change and decided I needed to be evaluated by a child psychologist. They told me the visit had been arranged because I was "fighting too much," or something along those lines, and I agreed to go. The reality was that I was not given a choice.

"Draw a picture of a boy your age and tell me all about his life." Give me a break, I thought, it's obvious that the person I draw is supposed to be me and that you want me to confess my deepest secrets. I questioned whether I should give the psychologist what he wanted or describe the life of someone totally opposite, just to mess with this guy I definitely didn't like.

After much internal debate, I decided to go with the opposite idea. Midway through, however, I began to panic. What if he believes that this degenerate I'm describing is me? I was sure he'd then recommend sending me away to school or even a military academy for kids with problems. A million concerns were now racing through my head.

From the drawing, we then moved on to the ink-blots, which were kind of fun. I described them all as monsters, since I loved watching Creature Features on television every Saturday night. Next was memorizing numbers; my task was to recite them backward and forward, given five, ten, fifteen at a time and more. Mentally, I was begging for something more challenging and couldn't believe how easy the remainder of the exams were as well.

All this testing lasted much longer than I had expected, but even worse, it was physically painful. It was almost summer, and with the air conditioner cranked to its highest level, the sterile office was freezing. I was in shorts and a tank top and kept drinking the water offered to me, which filled my bladder to the bursting point. The psychologist continually reassured me that the testing would soon be over and I would finally be allowed to use the restroom. I trusted that this torture was not an intentional part of the evaluation, but having had some exposure to unusual psychological techniques while in medical school, I now can't be so sure.

Thankfully, by the time the analysis wrapped up, I hadn't lost control of my bladder. I guess I passed the tests since I never returned to see the psychologist and I wasn't put on any medication. A few years later, I got up the nerve to finally ask my mother what this had all revealed. "It proved that you were a normal young boy," she told me. Maybe that was true, but something was going on regardless.

In the late sixties, "anything goes" was society's mantra. People commonly abandoned their responsibilities to "find themselves." Maybe this environment was acceptable for most kids, but I was in desperate need of direction and guidance in order to channel my energies in a positive manner. As I entered middle school, I was leaving a relatively innocent upper-middle-class neighborhood school to be thrust into a whole new world, one where kids were less fortunate and values were much different. We would soon be exposed to threatening pressures and given choices that could profoundly affect the rest of our lives. There would be no warnings, no advice, and certainly no preparation for what was to come.

Chapter Three:

WHAT A FINE
GROUP OF MEN

The students of Metuchen's three very different elementary schools came together in one middle school. My school, Moss Elementary, had been almost completely white and hadn't experienced racial controversy or significant violence. In Metuchen, white still meant minority, since we could all be divided into Catholics, Italians, Poles, Irish, Jews, Hungarians, and every possible combination. What the distinction really meant was that our elementary school had had few blacks and Puerto Ricans, groups that were prevalent at the other two grade schools. Kids from my school had been teased about being spoiled and from the rich side of town, which certainly wasn't true. However, it was unusual for Moss School families not to have both parents living under the same roof and a father with a steady job.

There was no formal orientation or introduction to Franklin Middle School, and on the first day as sixth graders, we walked in the front door and did our best to find our classrooms. Many of us were shocked by the diversity we encountered. These kids look and act really different, I thought. I had never personally known anyone with a 'fro before that time, but in 1969 the popular style for black kids was to tease out their hair to decent heights. Most of the black kids and later the white kids, including me, had huge combs we called picks hanging out of our back pockets for those moments when we might need to organize our mess. On occasion, picks made of metal were used as weapons.

The black kids in our school were not in the majority, but they definitely defined the culture. I experienced profound insecurity in this foreign environment and was overwhelmed by the confidence that followed this mentally and physically tough group. From the music to the attitude to the athletic ability, I was envious of what I witnessed and secretly questioned why I wasn't lucky enough to have been born black.

Behind this school were two full-length basketball courts with rims that rarely had nets. For durability, the few nets that did exist were not nylon but metal chain, which we all hated. Instead of the deeply satisfying swish when a perfect shot soared through without hitting the rim, you'd only get a jangle. The backboards were also metal, which made bank shots difficult because of the dead areas. The court had permanent lines drawn for out of bounds, half court, the foul line, and the lane. There were no three-point shots in those days, although that didn't discourage any of us from shooting from very far out. However, what made this court special and a magnet for the most talented players in the surrounding towns were the lights that switched on automatically after sunset. This unusual asset boosted our skills way more than we could have appreciated at the time.

First bell rang at 8:30, yet the courts were usually filled with pickup games by 7:30. We were allowed thirty minutes for lunch, but after squeezing in one or two games (and working up the rancid stench typical of adolescent boys), we barely had time to eat before rushing back to class. The games continued after school and well into the night.

Any time you'd arrive at the court, you'd yell, "I got next," and then pick four other players from the crowd to complete a team to challenge the winner of the game in play. It was always winner stays on, meaning you continued to play until you lost. If your team was good enough, you might play all night without ever sitting down. However, if your team was not especially talented, you'd spend two or three hours at the playground while getting in only a few games, which we felt was a waste of time. If you didn't have skills, you were rarely picked to play, which was cruel and humiliating. There wasn't anything remotely fair about this process, but we all understood that you got nothing for losing. It was always about competing and being the best.

Metuchen was a town of sixteen thousand residents squeezed into a few square miles. Even without a large population of kids to draw from, the popularity and attraction of basketball was tremendous. This could be attributed to the work of Coach Bill Blindow, a legend in our town, especially for the kids who played the game. Coach Blindow was a trim, crew-cut, no-nonsense individual; attributes unique for the time. Maybe he was out of step with the late 1960s, but in many ways he was exactly what the kids, many lacking direction, needed. He was the sole gym teacher for the Franklin Middle School boys, as well as the highly successful head coach of the Metuchen High School varsity basketball team.

Coach Blindow started each hour-long daily gym class by lining us up in military fashion, at full attention with our eyes straight ahead. Talking in line was a bad idea unless you were hoping for a quick trip to the principal's office.

"What a fine group of men" was his opening statement every day as we eagerly awaited our orders. Coach Blindow was a disciplinarian, but he cared more about developing our character. He also taught us the fundamentals of basketball from the first day we walked through his gym door—and taught it the right way.

Most of us had played some before, but the game had taken on no particular importance. My experience was on neighborhood rims attached to garages, often at severe angles to the ground, as driveways tended to slope toward the road. My own hoop sat on a pole stuck in the uneven grass in my rocky backyard. The basket was anywhere from nine to eleven feet high depending on where you stood (normal is a very precise ten feet). It wasn't much fun trying to dribble across a surface covered with dirt and stones to shoot at an eleven-foot hoop, but this was often all that was available to most of us.

Coach Blindow was a tremendous instructor. He held clinics on Saturday morning, and leagues went on throughout the week for most of the year. As you can imagine, after three years of this intense instruction, we arrived at high school with finely honed fundamental skills.

I don't know if Coach Blindow planned it this way or if being an instructor at Franklin School was simply an available job, but if it was deliberate, it was genius. He instilled in us the sense of challenge, the purpose, and the discipline that most of us so sorely needed at that time in our young lives. In addition, his job at Franklin School allowed Coach Blindow to develop some great players who would go on to lead his winning teams in high school. Many of his commands still echo in my brain today:

"Shoot the ball and always follow through."

"Dive for those loose balls."

"Block out your man."

"Dribble with your eyes up."

"See the entire court when handling the ball."

Early on in my initiation to the middle school hierarchy, I learned that those who played basketball were at the top. The playground stands surrounding the courts were generally filled with kids listening to music, talking trash, or just hanging out and watching the games. If you made a special shot before school or at lunch, word got around, so you got your proper respect as you walked between classes: "Nice move, Bruce," or "Great shot today, man." The opposite was true—for example, if you had your shot blocked well into the stands in front of a whole crowd, you would hear about that embarrassing and fortunately rare event for what seemed like months.

Basketball became my focus, and without my knowing it then, it filled many of my needs. As a result, sometime within the first few months of starting sixth grade, I made myself a silent promise that I took to heart:

By the beginning of my final year at Franklin School, I will be the top point guard of my class.

It sounds trite, but it was not an easy objective, considering that I had started nowhere near that level. Of greater significance than the promise itself was that this was the first time in my life I'd totally committed myself to anything important. I was quite certain that I would push harder than any other player to get there, and although I did not appreciate it at the time, it marked a major turning point. Basketball had given me not just the focus I desperately needed but the desire to achieve a goal.

* * *

With my textbooks and lunch in my left arm, I'd dribble my rubber Voit basketball right-handed to school in the morning. Going home from school, I'd switch off and dribble the whole way with my left hand. Every day I practiced the same routine during the two-mile walk. I realized that if I wanted to be a point guard, my ballhandling had to be second nature. I reasoned that the way to make the ball a part of you was to never be without it. I literally slept with the ball in my bed each night. Basketball was my passion, and no matter the time of year or weather, I played before, during, and after school. In the winter, I shoveled snow off the court to shoot several hours a day. Intense heat or rain was never a reason not to play. The playground was where I felt most at home, and by the end of my first year of middle school, I found myself part of the crowd that I had admired so greatly on those terrifying opening days. Basketball was our common denominator. To us, race or ethnic background didn't matter; you were judged only by your skills on the court.

My game was progressing well, but I thought I needed to develop even faster. To this end, Coach Blindow steered us all toward basketball camp. By reinforcing my skills and values, the experience would ultimately change the direction of my life.

Chapter Four:

TAKING IT TO
THE NEXT LEVEL

In the summer of 1971, I attended Dave Bing's All Pro Basketball Camp for the first of what would be four consecutive years. Bing was one of the elite NBA players at the time and an All-Star for the league, playing for the Detroit Pistons. My parents drove me up to the camp, located in the Pocono Mountains in Pennsylvania, several hours from Metuchen. Our first task was to drop off my gear at the assigned cabin. The no-frills room had windows with holes in the screens and accommodated six rickety double bunk beds to sleep eleven campers and a counselor. Dave Bing happened to be walking by at the same time I was checking into my bunk.

He graciously introduced himself, shook my parents' hands, and then looked at me and said, "Nice to meet you, Bruce. How old are you?"

"I'm fine," I said.

I'm fine? What was I thinking? I was completely overwhelmed meeting my first NBA star and assumed he'd ask, "How are you?" We eventually straightened it out, and I let him know I was thirteen. Having miserably failed his first appraisal, I was hoping that I would do better when it came to basketball challenges.

The next day, wake-up call blasted over the loudspeaker at 7:00 a.m. Most of us had been too excited to get much sleep, but we stumbled off to breakfast. Bing then lectured us on shot selection and movement without the ball, after which we were split into small groups with our counselors. For the next two or three hours, we practiced what we had learned. Lunch was followed by a rest hour and then more instruction. More drills and practice as well as league play was how we spent the last part of the afternoon. Every day followed this basic schedule.

League teams were organized by bunk and coached by our assigned counselors. In these games, we were able to try out the offensive moves and shots we had learned earlier in the day. The games were competitive, and more than anything we all wanted to end up in first place at the end of the week so we could take home a trophy, a difficult yet tremendously important feat.

Although these plastic awards were far from expensive, they represented something significant. Earning a trophy put you among the elite in a very talented group of campers. There were only two ways to win a trophy at camp: by being on the team that won first place in the league or getting named to the all-star team. Being chosen for this squad was difficult and, therefore, a real honor. It also meant you would eventually play a game at center court with the entire camp watching, including Dave Bing, who might serve as a referee. There were no trophies for second place and certainly nothing remotely resembling an award for participation.

It took me until my second year at camp to finally come home with a trophy. I had been chosen for the all-star team, but only as a substitute for an injured member of my squad. Chad Kinch from Perth Amboy, a rough town near Metuchen that had a tradition of producing tremendous athletes, was in the same grade as I was and played on my league team that summer. Over six feet tall already and with impressive skills from anywhere on the court, he certainly deserved the honor much more than I did, but he sustained an injury a day before the game and couldn't play. It wasn't exactly how I'd hoped to be chosen, but I was still pretty happy. Chad eventually went on to play for the University of North Carolina at Charlotte and was a first-round pick for the Cleveland Cavaliers in the 1980 draft. Missing that one game apparently didn't affect his career too much, and I was thrilled by the trophy, as it fulfilled another of my basketball goals.

Each day at camp, we worked on our games and played on the lighted courts until well after dinner. Exhausted from the twelve to fourteen hours of practice, we were never too tired afterward to secure a prime seat at center court for the chance to witness unparalleled basketball proficiency. The counselor games are among my favorite memories of camp.

Working for minimal compensation, the camp counselors were all active college players. These guys were not just any college players, however, they were standouts from traditionally distinguished and highly ranked programs. Many were considered top NBA prospects at the time, and during the school year we would read about them in the newspaper or see them on the cover of Sports Illustrated. They included Campy Russell from the University of Michigan, drafted number eight in 1974 by the Cleveland Cavaliers and later playing for the New York Knicks. Campy was present 24/7 and always happy to teach. Incredibly entertaining and upbeat, he was my assigned bunk counselor and the coach of our team one year. I got to know him fairly well and cheered him on from afar during his following season at Ann Arbor.

Other players of note were Rudy Hackett from Syracuse University, later drafted by the New Orleans Jazz; Terry Furlow from Michigan State, twelfth pick overall by the Philadelphia 76ers and noted mentor to Magic Johnson; Billy Ligon from Vanderbilt, drafted by the Detroit Pistons; and a very talented guard I considered my role model, Ed Iannarella, from a small basketball school in Pennsylvania, Lebanon Valley College. As an undersized point guard with a tremendous jump shot and incredible court sense, Ed had no problem running with the big boys and was eventually elected to his school's athletic hall of fame. His style of play was one that I patterned my own after, but more important, he helped me stay focused on my game and my priorities by setting a good example and keeping up with me during the school year. At a time when my buddies were routinely making poor choices, Ed's common-sense guidance helped keep me from making some of the same mistakes.

After a long day of instruction, Bing and the college stars were set to play five-on-five with standard playground rules and no referees. These evening games were what attracted all the great players to the camp and kept them coming back year after year. There was always a lot of trash-talking and intimidation;

the campers made a whole lot of noise, cheering for their favorite counselors. The level of play was phenomenal, and one could argue that these games were better than anything seen in college or the NBA. They were unadulterated playground ball with players who were among the top in the country. The big bonus was that these guys were able to work on their creativity without fear of being benched for an unorthodox decision or off-the-wall shot. The more innovative the display, the louder we yelled and cheered. It was all basketball and nothing else. We were thrilled and honored to be present, believing without any doubt that in the not-so-distant future, each one of us would be out there on that same court, playing at that same level of intensity and electrifying the campers in attendance.

For so many hours each day we were lectured on, drilled in, and inspired by basketball. Despite my throbbing legs from the nonstop play, each night I returned to my bunk with a huge grin, eager to take on the next day. I never felt more comfortable and didn't want to leave at the end of the session. If the playground was where I felt most at home, that feeling was tripled at camp. Finally, I was starting to understand who I was.

"What I Learned at All Pro Camp," dated July 31, 1971, is a fifteen-page booklet I put together after my first camp experience to record what I absorbed there. It outlines the drills for warming up, shooting, dribbling, and, most important, the "twenty-six offensive moves" as described by Coach Howie Landa, along with a few additions I made up. This book also highlighted instructional dogma that I learned from the coaches and players, which I often transferred to posters displayed prominently on my bedroom walls. One in particular influenced me more than the others:

Make Every Shot Count

That simple statement hung over my bed. It was the last image I took in before falling asleep and the first I saw when waking up. It meant that if a shot was worth taking, making that shot was worth the effort. I tried to apply this principle to my life in all ways. My thought was not to hope for success but to make success happen. I wonder if these guys had any idea how strong their influence was and how literally I took every word they uttered. By writing these words down and hanging this sentiment on my wall, I believed these ideals would become a part of me.

We learned defense well enough at All Pro Camp, but that was not the emphasis. To further advance this part of my game, I attended another camp later that summer, again with Coach Blindow's encouragement. This one was at West Point Academy, run by a young coach known for his discipline and defensive expertise, Coach Bob Knight. Although I was initially concerned about how the week would go, it turned out to be one of the most meaningful experiences of my young life.

After finding the building where I would stay, my parents dropped me off with little more than a "Have fun and we'll see you next Sunday." From the moment I stepped out of the car, I could feel that this camp was completely different from Dave Bing's. First of all, we were housed in clean dorm rooms, not rustic bunks. The toilets were actually functional and the showers were spotless. In addition, the kids didn't carry themselves with the cockiness I was used to. Certainly this was my own interpretation, but most of the other kids looked uncomfortable and nervous.

As I settled into my room and hung out in the dorm hallway that first night, the older campers kept telling me how during the week I was going to run nonstop and never even touch a basketball. "Defense—that's all you'll practice; you'll be lucky if you get even one shot up all week." I was one of the youngest campers enrolled, and these guys seemed to enjoy getting to me. Of course, I was smart enough not to let on that they had accomplished their goal. I was never going to give them an edge they could use on the court in the days ahead.

My stomach was in knots before we started our first clinic in the morning, and I kept reassuring myself that these older guys were only giving me a hard time and it couldn't be that bad. I told myself over and over that it was only a week and I could do anything for one week. After breakfast, which I barely touched, we all met in the gym and were given several racks of basketballs to warm up with. I watched the other kids shoot to assess the competition, just like I would do on the playground. My first thoughts were that the group was much whiter than I was used to.

I know that's a racial statement, but I was referring to the style of play, regimented and disciplined, relying more on knowledge of the game than on natural talent. It's amazing what you can learn just watching others warming up, and from that point on, I wasn't intimidated. I knew I would be just fine and that it was going to be a good week.

We first heard lectures from Coach Knight on the defensive stance. From day one, he used me to demonstrate despite my lack of experience. He may have chosen me partly because I was one of the youngest in the gym and he wanted to make me feel at home. But I was also singled out because I was the only camper in 1971 with very short hair, similar to Coach Knight's style.

During the end of the 1960s, most kids had long hair, a symbol of rebellion and solidarity with their generation. Like anyone my age, I wanted to be in style, accepted by my peers and not stand out in any way, at least in terms of appearance. Before going off to basketball camp, however, I decided my normal-length hair should be just a little shorter. Since we would be outside in the hot sun most days, I thought that would help keep me cool. I also figured I could handle this task on my own. Big mistake.

Under my parents' bathroom sink, I found a cheap plastic manual trimmer that you simply ran against the grain to thin out your hair. I had no idea how old it was or when it was purchased, but it seemed perfect for a minor trim. I quickly became frustrated, however, because it didn't appear to be doing anything as I worked it against my scalp. Deciding it needed a new razor blade, I appropriated one from my father's medicine cabinet and inserted it in what I thought was the correct slot, but I didn't realize that the trimmer was adjustable for different hair lengths. I then ran the razor firmly across the center of my head and created a huge divot right down to the skin.

"Ahhhh!"

Screaming and in tears, I ran downstairs to my mother, frantically asking if there was anything we could do. She held back her laughter and promised to drive me to the barbershop the next day. That night, I kept waking up and feeling my head in hopes that this would all turn out to be a bad dream and that I'd get up the next morning and laugh about the strangeness of it all. When I got to the barber, he smirked and muttered, "Serves him right," and proceeded to shave off any remaining hair right down to skin level.

The style would be fine now, but back then I stood out completely. Kids I'd never met made fun of me nonstop. They'd sneak up from behind and rub my head to provoke a response. When asked why my hair was so short, rather than admit to my stupidity, I claimed to have a "scalp disorder" (where I came up with that statement, I have no idea). In the fall, with my hair still not completely grown out, Coach Blindow looked at my choice of hairstyle with approval, believing he had influenced my decision in some way. I left his thought unchallenged and took to wearing a hat off the court until my hair grew back.

* * *

"Just imagine you're out in the woods with your pants pulled down to take a dump, and you don't want to get anything on your heels. That's the position you need to be in. Now shuffle your feet to stay in front of your man." This was the stance Coach Knight asked me to demonstrate to the rest of the campers. As soon proved to be his routine, he then sent us off to our stations to practice with the counselors until he blew his whistle to call us back for another lecture.

We learned early on that with the first whistle, we had to run to the area where the upcoming talk would be held. With the second whistle, you needed to be seated around the circle or suffer the consequences and run laps. Nobody wanted to be embarrassed, and therefore if you were anywhere near the basket and heard the second whistle, you would dive headfirst into the pack of kids. Actually, it was really fun, and not wanting to run more than I had to, I dived a lot.

As I said, because I was younger and had a strong work ethic, Coach Knight took a personal interest in me. Or at least it seemed that way, and that made me push myself even harder. He learned my name for the week and constantly used me for examples and instruction, which gave me a lot of confidence. At the end of the session, I was chosen as one of the sixteen kids who would participate in the all-star game, despite my age. This contest took place in front of the entire camp, including Coach Knight. I don't think I played very well, but I was grateful and honored to have had the opportunity to participate.

Coach Knight taught us the fundamentals of basketball incredibly well, but even more important, he instilled a sense of discipline that would help my game tremendously. At the end of my camp experience, I put together a second booklet, this one titled, "What I Learned at Round Ball School," dated August 14, 1971. It focused on defense and outlined drills to practice. I ended by writing a quote hammered home to us: "Make your man work for every shot." I once again created a big poster that stayed on my bedroom wall throughout high school. In the short term, the skills this camp emphasized influenced my game greatly. Of even greater value was the accelerated work ethic we were taught, which would assist me in my future endeavors much more than I could have imagined.

My middle school teammates and I had worked hard on our games during the summer, and come fall, our notable improvement inspired Coach Blindow to create a team he called the Basketeers, a group of kids who practiced long hours and gave halftime performances modeled after the antics of the Harlem Globetrotters. Our basketballs were red, white, and blue, like the American Basketball Association (ABA) balls of the time, and our best and most entertaining routines involved spinning the ball on our fingers. I had spent hours on end in my basement learning how to spin the ball with proficiency and confidence; I also figured out how to spin the ball on a pen. Eventually we all learned to hold a pen in our mouths, which could be pretty tough on the teeth but was impressive to watch. One day I got an idea to saw off a broom handle and drill a hole in the top of it to hold a pen. With this concept, we could now spin the red, white, and blue ball on a red, white, and blue painted broomstick four feet above our heads. It looked pretty cool. The local paper wrote about us, which was a thrill for a bunch of eighth graders.

Without a doubt, the highlight of the Basketeers' season was performing at the University of Maryland during halftime of a great ACC matchup against Duke. We raised the money for Coach Blindow to charter a bus, and we stayed in the University dorms. After our halftime routine, kids ran after us for autographs, begging that we sign their programs. That evening we were able to see the Baltimore Bullets, who were playing nearby. We were allowed to sit at court level and even hang out with some of the pro players. I was thrilled, especially because the game had been a blowout.

To make conversation, I asked one of the Bullets how he had the energy and stamina to play so well night after night. Not a great question, but also not terrible considering I was a thirteen-year-old kid who had high basketball aspirations of his own. This NBA star looked at me with a straight face, chewing on the toothpick hanging from his mouth, and said, "Drugs, baby, we just use drugs." Even then, I realized his answer was not appropriate, but I also knew it was true. There were drugs all around us at that time, and I was disheartened to hear him verbalize how he used them. My choice was to focus on basketball. To this day, I'm fairly certain this player was just taunting me and even then I understood the importance of being a role model, whether you like it or not. Keeping focused and away from distractions was hard enough for us, and it would only get more difficult as we got older. I could have used his help, but luckily there were others who stepped in.

By the time I reached my last year of middle school, I had achieved many of my goals. Basketball had taken top priority in my life, and I had attained a level I was proud of. I was now the leading point guard in my grade and probably for the entire school. I wasn't about to lose that distinction. The memory of fulfilling my promise would serve me well in later years as I encountered obstacles much more difficult.

Chapter Five:

IT'S ALWAYS ABOUT RESPECT

By the end of eighth grade, my parents had built a small, self-contained basketball court in our backyard. There was one basket, and the court extended only out to just above the top of the key, but I loved the setup and would spend hours on end practicing my shot in what I considered my personal sanctuary. The court itself was concrete and had a single light that allowed practicing well into the night, which I'm sure the neighbors were not thrilled about. Shot after shot went up, often while I listened to Marv Albert call the play-by-play for the Knicks games over the radio. "DeBusschere from the corner—yesss!" It was a far cry from the sloped grass-and-stone area where I'd first been introduced to the game. Even though the court couldn't accommodate more than four players, it wasn't unusual for my friends to congregate at my house to get in some half-court action.

My parents tended to go out of town a fair amount, but they always left my brothers and me with a babysitter to keep us organized, fix our meals, and make certain that we went to school. We usually liked who they found, but at one point, a new sitter came to our house, and it's an understatement to say that it didn't work out well. This elderly lady we had never met before wasn't friendly and didn't seem to like us much from the start. As usual, a group of my friends were with me playing at my backyard court, two-on-two with winner stays on. I came inside for a drink of water, and this lady startled me by demanding, "Who are the colored boys in the backyard?" Amazed yet somewhat amused by the question, I coolly asked who she was talking about, claiming I didn't see anyone of a different color on the court. I then asked her to point out which boys she was talking about.

Outwardly annoyed, she said, "How can you not see that there are colored boys in your backyard?" I had no idea why it was so important to her (well, really I did), but obviously she wasn't happy about the situation. If she had used the N-word, I would have had no problem physically removing her from my home, but instead I repeated and defended my answer, which made her even more upset. She left the room and didn't speak to me for the rest of the week, which from my standpoint was perfect.

Back at the court, I relayed the story to my friends, and we all had a good laugh. For the next few days, I invited over every black kid I knew, just to get her even more excited. We all found it pretty funny and didn't mind tormenting her.

With basketball dominating our lives, my group had made it through middle school and into our early teens having survived the temptations typical of that age. Most of us found communication at home fairly nonexistent, and together we figured it all out. Early on, we realized the importance of making good choices, and it was not uncommon to witness the downfall of those with less foresight. Drugs were readily available in the mid-1970s, and you had to make a choice at a young age. This also applied to cigarettes. I never minded seeing overconfident competitors from other towns light up a cigarette before or after a game. "That's it, keep smoking," I thought, knowing that no matter how talented they were, there wasn't a chance they could keep up with me. I was pushing myself to be better, and it was unfortunate that those players couldn't be strong or smart enough to make the right choice. We all had temptation and pressure, and most knew the right thing to do. It was up to each of us to decide, and my friends and I tried to back each other up.

Most of the kids who hung at the courts were underprivileged, from broken homes, and minorities, mostly black. Adults were never around and police weren't nearby, so drugs were everywhere. Marijuana was most prevalent, but at times hash, pills, and other drugs were being used and distributed out in the open throughout our games. Drinking alcohol was

considered normal even among the decent, older players, and no one thought twice about downing a few
beers to hydrate after a long night. It wasn't hard to
buy alcohol since the legal drinking age was eighteen
then and liquor store clerks rarely bothered to check
an ID if you looked anywhere close to fifteen. This
was the world we were exposed to by age eleven, and it
was scary to realize that more often than not, making
the right decision depended on luck and not being in
the wrong place at the wrong time.

Family life wasn't easy for many of my friends, and
frequenting their homes humbled me. Often they
shared beds with up to three brothers, usually in the
open living room and rarely in their own bedrooms.
Parents lay around, drunk or drugged out and often
incoherent. I was warned not to wake them for fear
of repercussion. Once after asking to use the phone
at one of my buddies' houses, I had to sweep off hundreds of cockroaches to find the receiver and even
avoid rodents that scrambled into the wall.

Given these experiences, I thought my family was wealthy beyond belief, and this made me

appreciate my own opportunity. Because of our dramatically different home lives, my friends and I spent many days and nights hanging out at my house. It was not uncommon for these guys to call my mother "Mom" since she always made them feel welcome and offered them the encouragement and attention they often lacked in their own homes. Growing up could get rough for many of my buddies, and they knew that my house was always a safe haven when things got too out of hand. I didn't mind, and as a result, my upper bunk bed was constantly in use.

Violence was also commonplace on our playground. Since competition was fierce on the courts, tempers became heated and threats flew continuously. But unlike today, we never took these seriously and probably didn't need to. Fights happened regularly and most were quickly extinguished, yet in certain situations, they were necessary and expected.

On one hot summer night, our team was dominating the court. Even though I had just finished eighth grade, I was fortunate enough to have been picked up by a group of four kids several years my senior who arrived before me. They were all on the varsity squad at Metuchen High School. This was an important night in my progress; I was learning and gaining confidence in my play. As I quickly moved up the court, I caught the ball to the right of the top of the key and was ready to make my move to the basket. Pushing hard left with a crossover dribble and then strongly driving right by first flipping the ball behind my back, I blew by my man and leaped in for a right-handed layup. My coverage was several steps behind me, and as I jumped into the air, a second defender picked me up under the basket. Instead of trying to block my shot, he jerked his head down, got under my legs, and flipped me. I hit the pavement hard, landing on the back of my neck. At first, I was stunned by the impact, but once I determined that I wasn't injured, I let out a torrent of f-bombs at the player who had submarined me. Not only could I have ended up with a spinal-cord injury, but he had shown me incredible disrespect. Even though I knew this guy and we had never had problems in the past, I scrambled up as quickly as I could and threw a punch to his face, then tackled him to the ground. Our teammates finally broke it up.

"What are you doing, Bruce? I wasn't trying to hurt you, man. It just happened."

I didn't believe him, but even if I did, it didn't matter. After a foul like that, my response was expected, even though he was considered a friend.

On rare occasions, a player would step up the rhetoric after a rough outing or after having been embarrassed or disrespected. "I'll kill you! I'm going to get my gun. I'm gonna shoot you dead. You'll see." These threats were usually from kids from the surrounding, more violent towns such as Perth Amboy, New Brunswick, and Newark who had come to our playground for the lights and the competition. We usually laughed in their face, never giving it a second thought. "Yeah, sure, you got a gun. Go get it. We'll be here playing ball. We'll wait for you to come back." We never took off or even got worried. In fact, we would have thought it was pretty exciting if the guy did show up with a gun, but luckily that never happened. On occasion a knife was seen, but no one was ever cut, at least not while I was there. A lot of broken bottles were used in fights because they were easily accessible from garbage cans, but we didn't care about those, either. We were young and foolishly thought we were invincible.

On the playground, no one told us how we were supposed to act. We just understood that being tough was important not just in the moment but for the future as well, in order to establish and maintain a reputation. It was always about giving and showing respect, at least in a way we all understood. On at least one occasion later in my basketball career, I forgot this important rule, and our group was lucky to get home that day without being hurt.

The players I hung around frequently pursued the better competition in the area. There was little to no organized communication and certainly no cell phones, so finding these games was hit or miss. One night we heard about an open gym in Linden, New Jersey, a small, fairly tough town just down the Garden State Parkway and known for its great basketball teams. One of the older kids was able to drive, and we loaded up a car and found the place. Despite not knowing anyone there, I yelled per our usual routine, "I got next," and began to assess the competition. The play was decent but by no means out of our league, and we looked forward to establishing ourselves on the court. We'd brought a small but fast team and realized that the only way we could win was to continually run, playing the game in high gear.

We won our first game handily and stayed on the court for a second, only to go up against a team that seemed more interested in fighting than in playing ball. The guard covering me was particularly annoying, talking trash nonstop to cover up his lack of skills. I was having difficulty getting my shot off. He physically held me whenever I made a move to the basket, and I let him know I wasn't happy with his play. Finally, I'd had enough. Not only did I want to score on him, but I wanted to embarrass him as well.

As I was pushing the ball up the court on the left side, I found myself in a one-on-one break on him. I pushed the ball to my right hand as I approached the basket and held it out, essentially daring this guy to take it away. He took my fake, and I quickly moved the ball behind my back and went in for a soft layin. I had practiced this maneuver hundreds of times on my own on the playground but was rarely able to use it in a game. It turned out well—I got my team the basket and showed my opponent what I thought of him.

"Walk!" he screamed. We both knew I hadn't.

"No way," I said, at which point he got in my face and threatened to knock me out. My crew had my back, but we were way outnumbered and not near our home court. After a lot of threats, we elected to end the game early and leave, happy to find our car intact with no slashed tires.

No, I hadn't traveled with the ball, but I knew negotiating that move would get that reaction. I had shown my opponent complete disrespect, and he knew it. That's why I rarely tried to use this move in a game. That day I had lost my composure. I decided that I was going to shut this clown up by making him look bad on his own court in front of his boys. By demonstrating that he deserved no respect, I gave him only one option. His message was received loud and clear. We could now either stand and fight or leave the building, and we knew that it was a smart move to get out.

Basketball in general and the playground in particular taught me the importance of respect, an essential lesson I would carry with me for life.

Chapter Six:

THE REAL PURPOSE OF PLATFORM SHOES

Everyone wanted to be on Brad's team. We operated under the steady rule that winners stayed on, so if you were fortunate enough to be on Brad's team, you never sat out because you never lost. Brad Sellers had moved from Perth Amboy in seventh grade, and it was my good fortune that we were in the same year at school. Lightning quick and 6'2" by the time he started high school, Brad was unstoppable.

On the playground, teams were chosen in the usual manner, but no matter who showed up, if Brad was on the team, he would make sure that I was the next player chosen after him. Kids several years older and five to six inches taller than me would just shake their heads, make comments, and roll their eyes, wondering what I had done to deserve such distinction. For Brad, loyalty was very important, and I was lucky to be his friend. In reality, this arrangement worked well for both of us, since I was a true point guard and good at dishing out assists, while Brad was a terrific scorer. Eventually he became one of the few players in Metuchen High School basketball history to score more than 1,000 points, and I can't imagine how many assists I was credited because of his skills. At the Franklin School playground, we rarely lost, and I had the honor of playing daily with one of the best players I have ever known, including many I saw go on to NBA careers. I looked forward to playing with him at an even higher level of competition in high school.

In the fall of 1973, my freshman year had begun, and we were eager to test our skills against the area's best teams in organized competition. We had practiced our drills and shooting techniques nonstop, been to camps and clinics, and spent countless hours on the playground. From our perspective, tryouts for the freshman team were only a formality. We already knew who should be on the team and even who deserved to be in the starting lineup. We now had to demonstrate our skills to the freshman coach, Mike Costello, whom none of us had met.

For us, basketball season was 365 days a year, so we arrived at our first tryouts in great physical shape. If you weren't at our level of conditioning, by the end of the first session you'd find yourself over the trash can in a corner of the gym, vomiting from pain. That didn't happen much and only to those who had the audacity to show up without having put in the playground time. Our freshman team went on to have twenty-two wins and only two losses for the season. It was great fun, gained us recognition, and showed us that we actually were pretty good when put up against the surrounding towns. It was also critical for our development to truly understand the relationship between hard work and success. The experience helped many of us overcome insecurities typical of our age and certainly part of my makeup. I further appreciated there was never anywhere that I was happier than on the basketball court, whether at the playground, in my backyard, or in front of a screaming crowd of fans who had come to watch our game.

During my sophomore year on the junior varsity squad, our skills continued to improve, yet I realized that varsity was the only game that really mattered. Metuchen's varsity teams were exceptional. By this time, Brad was a star, and the varsity guys played to packed houses with good support from the student body. At the end of the season, they continued on to the state tournament. Coach Blindow asked me to come up to varsity for these games, a rare occurrence and a real honor for a sophomore. This allowed me to practice with the varsity or sit on the bench and cheer my teammates on—unless, of course, we were up or down by 40 points, and then I might get a few minutes of playing time. Even more important to me was that as a sophomore, I was assigned a varsity uniform. After receiving it, I pulled it on and stood in front of the mirror for well over an hour. I was excited and proud.

The varsity team was eliminated from the state tournament fairly early that year. With the season over, we had eight months to prepare for the next. I was ready to move up and knew that I would not be satisfied unless I was the starter; I didn't want to play backup to anyone despite this being the junior point guard's usual role. At that moment, I made a second silent promise:

I promise that I will be the starting point guard on the varsity team by early next season.

To be among the starting five, I knew I would have to push out a great player, Tommy Alicino, a rising senior who had spent the previous season at the backup position waiting for his opportunity to run the team. A junior point guard rarely started in Metuchen, so I would have to step up my game tremendously. I was ready to go back to Dave Bing's camp, this time as a junior counselor. It was only the end of February, and I couldn't wait for summer.

At All Pro Camp, being a junior counselor meant I attended for free in exchange for assisting the counselors with teaching drills and helping run the camp. My assignment was to scrub the showers and clean the toilets in the community area every day—not glamorous and at times pretty disgusting, but I did my job without complaining.

I lived in a bunk with eleven other junior counselors, and we had our own highly competitive league. Since Dave Bing played for the Pistons, the other junior counselors were mostly from the Detroit area and were rumored to be from some pretty rough neighborhoods. I was the only white guy in the mix, but this was inconsequential since my bunkmates couldn't have cared less. As always, the hierarchy and the acceptance came from the skills. I was happy around these guys and as an added bonus, the nonstop music blaring from our radios and tape players was tremendous. These kids were from Motown, and it was 1974. The music didn't get any better than that.

As a junior counselor, I had more time to hang out and listen to the counselors' stories about playing college ball in front of packed arenas and in televised, high-pressure games. Even more entertaining was listening to Bing and his peers tell their stories from the NBA. On one occasion, I was invited to go to a restaurant with most of the college players, Dave Bing, and Bob Lanier, a 6'11" teammate of Bing's who had been at the camp instructing that day.

I sat at a huge table with these guys, loving every minute as I listened to their stories, each trying to outdo the others. I was fully confident the day would come when I'd have my own stories to tell. It was a great summer, and my game had again developed to another level completely.

Back at Metuchen High School, junior year, basketball practice started November 15. I had given myself until Christmas to become a starter. I lived by the rule that you improve your game in the off-season and earn your playing time during practice. I knew I had worked hard enough to be a part of the starting lineup, and now it was up to me to prove myself on the court. As a result, the first month of practice became an all-out war between me and the senior point guard. As much as I truly liked and respected Tommy, I wanted to hurt him, not in a bad or unsportsmanlike manner but in as competitive a way as possible. Any loose ball I dived for; any scoring opportunity I took. I used every bit of defensive knowledge I had learned from Coach Knight to contest every shot. If I fouled Tommy, it was just too bad. Nothing was going to come easy for anyone in my way. Most likely, those battles improved both of our games, which ultimately could do nothing but help the team.

One day around Christmas, Coach Blindow announced that I had been assigned to the starting lineup—side by side with Tommy. Coach decided to start two guards instead of one, and teamed with two 6'7" big men as well as Bradley, our leading scorer, we had a pretty tough squad. I'd kept my second promise to myself, and I was flying high.

"I'm not sure how you can even get that big head of yours through the door," one of my closest friends often said. I didn't mind, for this confidence would help save me in later years when things weren't going so well. It felt great to work so hard and, as a result, realize a dream.

With the season in full swing, we were required to "dress to represent your school" on game days. In the 1970s, this meant a collared shirt, wide bell-bottom pants, and nice shoes, not sneakers. The shoes, strategic enhancements of our attire, were mostly very high platforms. Originally designed for the disco scene and popular for a short time, these shoes served a very different function for our team. With heels up to five inches, we calmly moved into the opposing gym, our game faces in place, trying to appear as threatening as possible. With the extra inches attributed to our footwear, two of our starting five would come in somewhere around 7'0", one at 6'7", another at 6'3", and yours truly at 6'1", making our team's size daunting. We knew exactly what we were doing.

Warmups were intended for loosening up and getting comfortable, but for our team this practice provided another opportunity to gain an edge. At that time, dunking the ball wasn't allowed in either high school or college games, but that didn't stop us from showing off in the pregame layup drills. Moving quickly to the rim, we would jump high with the layin and on the way down, slap the fiberglass with a loud crack. The backboards were usually square, extending low toward the floor, allowing even me, the smallest member of the squad, to show off in this way. Our attitude was to always look cool, act confident, and stare into your opponent's eyes. Search for that fear, and don't ever be the first to blink.

That year, I hung a sign to the side of my bedroom desk: "Success is 90% in your Head." I understood that if you don't truly believe you can beat your opponent, you won't. As a team, we knew that we had the skills to beat anyone, but we figured we might as well start before the opening buzzer. The coaching staff never encouraged our actions, but then again, we were never asked to stop.

As I moved along in high school, my successes on the court meant a lot to me, certainly a great deal more than anything else. Even through my junior year, I still rarely took home a book to study, and my classes, which were by no means accelerated, continued to earn me As and Bs, with the occasional C. By this time, I knew I wanted to attend college but really just to play ball. When it came time to take the SAT,

I thought it was reasonable to listen to recommendations and study for it.

When I attended my high school's first SAT prep class, I was given a very large practice book. We were all instructed to try some sample questions to establish our weaknesses. I barely got a single answer correct, so I quickly became discouraged with my poor performance and determined that this first class was to be my last. I decided I wasn't going to waste my time studying for the exam, rationalizing that the SAT really didn't matter much. I was sure that I could do well enough on the SAT to get into a school where I could play ball.

In the middle of my junior year, I sat in homeroom as one of my more academically competitive classmates loudly complained about earning a B in gym class. I couldn't understand why anyone would even care about gym class, and after all, a B wasn't that bad. I was compelled to ask why the grade mattered so much to him.

"It messes up my GPA."

"GPA?" I said.

"Your grade point average."

"Huh?"

"The average of all your grades. For colleges to look at," he said condescendingly.

"They actually keep that?" I asked. I now marvel at my naiveté and how little I prioritized grades.

I eventually did take the SAT on schedule. And although I never did attend another preparatory class or study for the test, I did well on the exam, so well that I now could think about attending some highly competitive colleges. The new information changed a lot about how I saw myself, and for the first time in my life, I began to think that maybe, contrary to what I had been led to believe for so long and by so many people, I was bright after all.

Chapter Seven:

READY TO MOVE ON

I don't know that any one incident brought it about, but by my senior year of high school, I found myself changing a lot. Maybe I was finally growing up, but now I was starting to think about who I was and the person I wanted to become. To disrupt my world further, Coach Blindow decided to move on to bigger opportunities coaching at Rutgers University, and I wasn't sure what role basketball would play in my life or in the future. For the first time in a long while, I found myself out of my comfort zone, even though it was my last year of high school and I should have been cruising along unhampered. If that wasn't enough for a seventeen-year-old, now I had the police after me as well.

It was always believed among the kids that I grew up with, that the police of our small town had some type of drug file or a list of suspects involved with narcotics. And all of a sudden, it was obvious that I was somewhere near the top of that list. Sure, a number of my friends were heavily into the drug lifestyle and supported their own habit by dealing. These were neighborhood kids I'd known since grade school, so I wasn't about to forgo them. But for whatever reason, my life became very complicated almost overnight.

I had a driver's license but no car, so my usual mode of transportation was on foot. I can tell you that being on the drug list made walking around town a real adventure. Often, when the police drove by in their squad cars and identified me, I was stopped and searched. "Keep your hands visible. Get on the ground, facedown." And then I'd be patted down, warned, and told to go on my way. This same drill occurred a number of times that year, and instead of reporting these unquestionable harassments and illegal searches, I usually mouthed off to the officer and laughed about it later with my friends. I wonder how I was never beaten up or at least arrested. This whole affair didn't faze me mostly because I didn't appreciate the inherent danger. Knowing the rules of this new game, I simply tried to play things smart and never give the police a reason to take me into custody. On most occasions, the officer would not have found anything incriminating on me. But not always, especially one careless evening where my life may have taken a very different direction.

I was walking up Main Street when a buddy asked me to hold some liquor for him. So I shoved the bottle of Jack Daniel's deep into the pocket of the long coat I usually wore. Less than one year from legal drinking age, I wasn't too concerned about getting caught. Alcohol was at every party we attended. In fact, it was so prevalent most of us didn't even think of it as illegal. At about eleven o'clock that frigid winter night, a police officer spotted me with a few friends walking toward the middle of town. He must have seen something suspicious or recognized me because he quickly swung his squad car around and flipped his siren on. I knew what was coming next, and this time I panicked. I didn't believe underage alcohol possession was a serious offense, but I didn't want to go to jail or have anything on my record. What would have hurt the most, though, was that being arrested might have had me thrown off the team.

There was only one officer in the car, and noting his poor physique, I knew if I ran that he would never catch me. "Freeze!" he yelled as he slammed on the brakes and jumped out of his car. This time, as I heard the familiar command, I followed my instincts and ran like hell.

I cut through backyards and between houses as I ran home, tossing the bottle along my route. Because I grew up in this small town, I knew exactly which yards were fenced in (and even which ones had holes in the fences), which had shrubs, and where to turn or not to turn. Eventually I made it home, expecting the police to pound on the door at any moment. I didn't feel relieved until after a week had passed without a visit. This time I had no one to blame but myself for being careless.

Having friends involved in illegal activities often made my life inconvenient, but there were other times it benefited me. During my early teens, my parents bought me a decent bicycle for getting around. My orange 10-speed Schwinn was reliable and sturdy, and if I wasn't on foot, this was how I got around. Yet despite being careful, it was stolen two times in high school. You have to realize that if your bicycle was taken in a small town like Metuchen, you could pretty well guess who the guilty party was, but accusing them might bring you harm. I was lucky that each time my bike was stolen, I simply contacted a friend and his response would be, "Don't worry, Bruce, I'll take care of this for you." By the next day the bike was delivered in good condition directly to my front door, no questions asked. It paid to have friends with all kinds of interests.

Senior year was moving along quickly, and despite our team's talent, the season turned out to be less than stellar. Bradley was racking up tremendous statistics with his scoring prowess and would eventually be chosen for conference honors, but with Coach Blindow no longer leading us, our overall record was mediocre.

Toward the end of the season, we played a rival team that we should have dominated due to its absence of height in the front court and lack of quickness at the guard position. I was playing horribly, as was the rest of the team. With little time left in the game, we were down by more than 20 points.

At this time, the outcome was already decided by the score, yet I missed an easy shot and fell hard to the floor, landing on the opposing guard. This guy had played well and had shut me down completely. I knew I was a better player than he was, but not on this night. With the ball now at the other end of the court, my defender and I started to get back to our feet. The appropriate action would have been for me to offer a hand to help him up. But I was so sick of his disciplined play making me look foolish that as I got up, I instead took the opportunity to step on his chest. He reacted just as I would have: he threw a punch to my face. And I returned the favor. My buddies in the stands ran out onto the court in my defense, pounding my opponent and then going after his teammates.

Both teams in their entirety joined the fight, which was now on the verge of turning into an all-out riot. Fortunately, security was quick to respond, and order was restored without serious injury. I was charged with two technical fouls, ejected from the game, and escorted by the police out of the building. In reality, I was happy to be put out of my misery.

As this was a Friday night game, I was well aware that I would have to wait until Monday to find out if there would be any further repercussions. For now, I was more concerned about the next morning's practice, where we were sure to hear a whole lot about our play.

"Keep running. I'll let you know when I'm ready for you to stop. You guys make me sick. I don't even want to look at you." We ran around the gym for at least forty-five minutes before our coach finally called us over to review the previous night's play. He broke down the entire game for us with an assortment of adjectives such as embarrassing, awful, and dreadful. He finally singled me out with the word horrendous. Still in a lousy mood over my performance and complete loss of control during the game, I leaned over to one of my teammates and asked, "Did he say horrendous or tremendous?" Unfortunately, the coach heard the comment, which bought me a whole lot more running time. At that moment, I just didn't care. It had been a rough couple of days.

Monday morning I was called to the principal's office. I waited outside on an overstuffed Naugahyde chair to discuss my role in the incident. My imagination had run wild all weekend, mostly because my friends kept giving me grief about school suspension and community service. Some even brought up the possibility of jail time. I'm sure they didn't actually believe I'd end up in prison, but the guys were enjoying the fact that they were starting to get to me.

When I was finally called in to see the principal, he was friendly enough and asked me to explain exactly what had happened. Luckily, he had not attended the game or seen any footage since there were no recordings back then. I described the exchange and emphasized that it's always the retaliatory punch that gets noticed, which was actually true if one ignored the part where I stepped on my opponent's chest. I wasn't proud of my actions, but I wasn't overly ashamed, either. For one moment, I had forgotten that I couldn't play in organized basketball the same way I'd played on the playground. I was lucky that the principal had once been a ballplayer himself and had always liked me.

"Don't let it happen again, Bruce."

"Yes, sir."

Years later, I found out that indeed the police were considering charging me with inciting a riot, since so many people were involved due to my actions on the court. Because I had not been arrested before, though, they agreed to let the principal handle the discipline. My life may have taken a much different course if that weren't the case.

Toward the end of my senior year, my focus started to change drastically. I began to appreciate the importance of academics, and for the first time, I took an advanced class. As I sat in this higher-level science course, I felt completely out of place. To make matters worse, the so-called intellectuals ridiculed me. I couldn't believe it. These were the same students obsessed with college admissions and GPAs. They ran for student government or joined student organizations just so it would "look good on their applications." I didn't do any of those things, so my presence was perceived as odd. Some went out of their way to make me feel as if I didn't belong. There were even teachers so convinced I was a dumb jock that when I handed in a high-quality paper, they accused me of plagiarism. These attitudes, combined with my own intellectual insecurities, made for a less than pleasant classroom experience.

"That's a stupid answer," one of my presumably gifted classmates said about my response to a teacher's question in my first accelerated class. I imagine I wasn't supposed to hear that remark, and it upset me greatly. My mother suggested I meet the guy after school and smack him around or at least threaten to hurt him. I was shocked—I thought she wanted me to get past that behavior, but I understood her sentiments. Fortunately, I didn't take her advice and instead just let this incident and others go. I was friendly with some intimidating people, so if it came down to it, I knew I could ask for a favor like injuring an easy target. They wouldn't have passed up the opportunity.

* * *

At the time, one of my closest friends had an older sister at Northwestern University. She encouraged me to at least check into applying there. I'd never heard of Northwestern, because most of the kids I knew who had gone on to college had been steered toward small schools in Pennsylvania. Many of my peers played ball for these colleges, and in the beginning of my senior year, that was my expectation as well. But hearing about Northwestern stirred my interest, and I decided to visit with my dad.

Walking on the campus, with Lake Michigan on its eastern border, I was overwhelmed and excited about the opportunities a large university would afford me. Having grown up outside New York City, I appreciated the benefits of being near a city the size of Chicago. Even as an undergraduate, I would have access to a whole range of activities. Almost overnight, basketball became less important to me. I was ready to push myself harder than ever, this time academically.

So I applied to Northwestern. As part of the application process, I was required to compose an essay describing how my life experience related to my future goals. Because I hadn't learned to type, I handwrote my essay about growing up on the playground, the lessons I had learned from it, and my ability to relate to people of all backgrounds and intellectual capacities. I talked about never forgetting where I had come from and using those rich experiences for whatever my future would hold. The essay was honest and unpretentious, and I believe it was part of why I was accepted to the school as an early admission. I am certain that many applicants more qualified than me could, and maybe should, have been admitted in my place, but I realized that I had been given a fantastic opportunity and planned to make the most of it.

If there was one thing I had learned from growing up on the playground and excelling in basketball, it was how to compete—never for anything less than first place. This sense of competition, drilled into my very being, influenced me as I made my third promise just before going off to college:

* * *

I promise that I will push myself harder than ever, and this time in academics.

With that in mind, I was ready to pack up my life and move to Evanston to begin my freshman year at Northwestern University. The last season had pushed my basketball passion to the side; being average wasn't much fun, especially when we had the potential to achieve greatness. Though Bradley had a tremendous year on the court and earned a number of accolades, his skills would not be enough to take him to the college level due to his poor academic record and lack of guidance.

Though I was ready to move away from Metuchen to attend college, I had no idea how unprepared I would find myself once I got there.

Chapter Eight:

IN WAY OVER MY HEAD

Almost overnight, my confidence became over-inflated. I'd graduated from high school, and when Northwestern sent out a questionnaire inquiring about preferences for a major, I chose premed. I'd decided I wanted a career in science, and being a doctor was something I could get really excited about. Certainly, I wasn't convinced I had the intellect to ever get into medical school, but I was ready to put my last promise to the test.

I arrived at campus in September 1976. As I got to know my classmates, it became painfully obvious that I was starting at a real academic disadvantage. For example, I found my entry-level calculus class almost hopeless. From the first day, the curriculum moved rapidly, but the explanations given in lectures weren't comprehensive. No one else seemed bothered by this manner of teaching; in fact, most of my classmates considered this course an easy A since they'd taken high school calculus. For them, this was just a review, and the fact that I didn't have the background to keep up was not my professor's concern. The same held true for a number of my other classes. To make matters worse, I had no idea how to study or even budget my time since these disciplines weren't part of my high school routine. I began to worry about the possibility of flunking out of Northwestern and begging for a new college to accept me.

The students came mostly from the Midwest, and a large number had been high school valedictorians or salutatorians. Many informed me that they'd always dreamed of going to Northwestern, which pushed them to focus on their studies early. It was not uncommon for these bright, multitalented kids to be recruited by several prestigious colleges. My closest friend was an accomplished musician, had earned almost perfect SAT scores, and was valedictorian of

his high school, having received only one B throughout all four years. You could tell how painful it was
for him to relate that "breakdown" (the shameful,
single B!) despite its minimal implications. Of course,
I would never have dared inform him of the plethora
of C's that had graced my final high school transcript.

If competing with the standard Northwestern student wasn't hard enough, I also had candidates from a
six-year medical school program in my premed classes.
These kids were recruited for their intellect with the
promise that they would attend undergraduate college
for only two years before going directly to medical
school for four. This meant they'd earn both a bacca-
laureate in science and a doctor of medicine in only six
years. So among this group of students, I tried my best
to earn A's, which were awarded to a fixed percentage
of each class since we were graded on a curve. This
manner of evaluation meant that a defined number of
my classmates would get an A (10 percent), a defined
number would get a B (20 percent), and this went on.
So if the person next to you earned an A, you had less
chance of achieving that same grade. Despite recog-
nizing the intensity of this grading system, I decided

to go full force. There was no way that I was going down without a fight.

My first quarter, I took the most difficult freshman course: inorganic chemistry. In fact, it was such a difficult class that it often convinced premed students to change their major. The course's mammoth lecture hall held more than two hundred students. My first test returned a C minus, which upset me, but I wasn't shocked or devastated. I appreciated where I was starting from, and if basketball had taught me anything, it was how to move from a poor performance and on to the next challenge. With this suboptimal grade and the others that followed shortly thereafter, I focused by thinking back to my days at Franklin Middle School and my efforts to become a top point guard. Whenever I was struggling in class, I reminded myself, "I've been here before. This is the same as figuring out basketball."

The first few months tested my resolve. I made B's and C's—nowhere near the almost perfect average I needed to get into medical school. As discouraged as I became at times, I never thought about quitting. Eventually, I established a study routine: five days a week I'd go to the library, arriving by 7:00 p.m. after a full day of classes and not leaving until it closed at 2:00 a.m. More time was spent on Saturdays and Sundays. These long hours were necessary to catch up from what I hadn't been taught in high school. The only problem was that I had no time for any other activities. I missed playing ball and began to question my decision to attend a large university and not continue that other aspect of my life. After all, I had essentially stopped playing ball cold turkey, assuming it had to be academics or time on the court. It wasn't until after a full year of playing catch-up with my academics that I finally realized I could compete academically with anyone. My focus and drive was unprecedented, thanks to the countless hours I spent in an isolated library cubicle cultivating the skills I'd found completely unnecessary in high school. I would love to say that there were never any setbacks, but that wasn't the case. After all, I was still only eighteen years old, and despite my heroic efforts, the necessary challenge of studying seven to ten hours a day left me tired, or perhaps restless is a better term.

In the first week of my second quarter, I received a phone call from my friend Ray, a close buddy from Metuchen High School. He wanted to visit me on his way to Navy boot camp at Great Lakes. It was a perfect opportunity to let loose with someone I felt totally comfortable with. I knew that I was changing, but I hadn't suppressed my old self completely. I missed being a big fish in a small pond, receiving recognition as I walked down Main Street in Metuchen. I felt nondescript at Northwestern, just another freshman enrolled in entry-level classes, with high ambitions that may or may not ever materialize. If I was to succeed, I knew I couldn't allow myself the luxury of self-doubt. But on those dark nights in the stacks of the library, uncertainties crept in.

The legal drinking age in Illinois was eighteen, and since none of us had cars, our transportation to the bars was by taking the elevated line into Chicago. Not driving was a good thing. There were no public service announcements reminding people to always have a designated driver. With that in mind, Ray, my roommates, and I jumped on the train to get to

Howard Street, a haven lined with dive bars surviving off Northwestern students on their almost daily pilgrimages from Evanston, which at the time was a dry town.

The night went as planned. We talked about old times and dreams for the future, but more important, we drank a whole lot of beer, as freshman boys are expected to do. When last call came, we were ordered to leave the bar, so we stumbled back to the station and waited for our train. By this time, our group had grown to more than fifteen freshman guys happy to be back at college after Christmas break and once again without home curfew. This collection of testosterone-engorged teenagers was not ready for the night to end, if only because we understood it meant getting back into the high pressure of freshman classes. As we walked down the street and approached our dormitory, one of my roommates noted a parking meter tilted at a 45-degree angle in a small parking lot on the side of a bank. It must have been knocked over by a car backing out.

"Hey, that would look great in our room, wouldn't it, guys? Let's see if we can pull it up," someone yelled.

A prolonged and boisterous "Yeeeaaaah!" was the overwhelming response from the gathering of intoxicated disciples. My roommate was able to persuade several others to pull the meter out of the ground and carry it up to our room to join the other "conversation pieces" he'd collected over the previous few months. As we were passing the bank's large storefront window, somebody then got the idea to throw the meter through the plate glass "just for some fun." Now, this was getting really stupid.

I only partially heard this conversation, so it didn't completely register until the yelling began. When I heard "one and two and ...," I knew I had better jump in. Running at full speed, I yelled, "Nooooooooo," and grabbed the heavy metal battering ram, pushing my friends away and hanging on to it for dear life to be sure it went no farther. My heart was beating out of my chest when three squad cars with flashing red lights descended on us, accompanied by screeching tires.

"Freeze!" six police officers with guns drawn yelled in succession. The four of us, still holding the meter, quickly dropped it and held our arms high in the sky. I saw one of my roommates thrown against the squad car face first and handcuffed in a single motion. The other two were treated the same way. Somehow I pulled a female officer, who put on my cuffs lightly and gently placed me in the squad car while shielding my head.

Ray was dragged into the whole mess through no fault of his own, and I wondered how the Navy would view his getting arrested before boot camp even began. Yet he found the whole situation pretty funny. Our friends who were lucky enough not to have been carrying the meter scattered in all directions at the first sound of the sirens. That was the group I tended be in, but this time I was cuffed and taken for a ride.

When we arrived at the police station, still under the influence of the pitchers of cheap beer, we had yet to fully appreciate the gravity of the situation. First, we were ordered to have our pictures taken, and we all worked hard to look as mean as we could for our mug shots. After all, that's something you want to show your grandkids someday (or maybe not).

* * *

After that our fingerprints were taken. Still not thinking straight, my roommate used his one allowed phone call to order a pizza, or at least he tried to, but by then our favorite delivery kitchen was long closed. The police did not find this amusing, and by this point I wasn't happy either. Upon being processed, we were left in a holding area, where we heard over and over from a fellow detainee speaking to the guard outside the cell, "Officer, what we have here is a simple case of mistaken identity." We laughed at him from the cell and repeated this line for months around our suite afterward. Somehow, it never got old.

After calling our friends (actually, the same guys who had been with us earlier), we were able to post bail and be released, just in time to get in a few hours of sleep. When we all eventually woke up, heads pounding and ink staining our hands, nothing was quite so funny anymore. Shit! After everything I had been through growing up, all the close calls and times I mouthed off to the police, I couldn't believe I'd been busted for something this stupid. Thank goodness I'd been successful in stopping the real intent of these guys. I imagine breaking into a bank would have kept us in that jail a whole lot longer.

We did have to hire a lawyer and ultimately had our day in court. The judge was understanding but didn't find the prank funny. With all the fraternities on campus, he may have been used to dealing with Northwestern kids doing stupid things. He eventually threw the case out with a small fine, calling it a misdemeanor, but he warned us that if he'd decided to count the money in the meter as part of the theft, it would have been a felony. (Potential felony number three for those keeping score.) We were never sure if this threat was true, but we all eventually had our records cleared without an overwhelming financial investment since we used a young lawyer.

This experience taught me a lot. I knew I had changed from my days in Metuchen, and I realized that if I were to succeed in college and beyond, it was essential to leave much of my old life and values behind. I knew I wasn't going to slip up again. It was time to grow up.

* * *

The first year at Northwestern proceeded with no further setbacks, and I started to do well in my classes, actually very well. I finally felt like I belonged at the school and was hopeful that my period of adaptation and initial low grades would not keep me out of the running for medical school. By sophomore year, I was on a positive streak, enrolled in hard-core science courses and routinely earning A's—that upper 10 percent. I had figured out what was necessary to excel and was starting to feel comfortable with academics and, even more important, with myself. My junior and senior years continued in the same manner, and my overall college experience was positive.

When graduation approached, I realized how much I owed Northwestern. I had been inspired to work hard and cultivate my academic skills to be able to compete with anyone. Because I had learned to study in a disciplined manner, I was well prepared to go on to medical school with the confidence I needed to make it through those even more demanding studies. Now, however, I wasn't so sure I could get any medical school to accept me since my grades were at the lower edge of accepted candidates. As I submitted my application to each medical school, I said a little prayer in hopes that someone would give me a chance. I knew I could do well; I just needed the opportunity to prove myself.

Chapter Nine:

BETTER OFF
BECOMING A RABBI

When you're checking the mailbox each day for a medical school acceptance letter, you quickly learn that a thin envelope is not a good sign. After receiving a whole lot of rejections from private medical schools, I finally received an invitation for an interview at the state medical school in New Jersey, which was where I had the highest chance statistically of being accepted. On a wet, dreary spring day, I took a direct flight to Newark from Chicago, feeling positive about my chances. For two years at Northwestern, I had been involved with research in basic cell biology that had been published. I'd even spent extra time in the summers and during the school year working as a phlebotomist, drawing blood to get some experience with patient contact. I hoped the extra effort would help distinguish my application and demonstrate my commitment.

Visiting applicants were first given guided tours, usually by upper-level medical students who would brag about the low number of students per cadaver in anatomy lab and go on about their facility's CT scan, which at that time was a new, expensive technology and something to be proud of. Because the admissions process was so competitive, all we cared about was getting accepted, but we still tried to look impressed and interested as the facts were relayed. In reality, we understood that it probably didn't matter where you went to medical school; any American medical school would deliver a quality education, since the curriculum was nationally standardized.

After the tours, I arrived at the admissions building, excited and enthusiastic about having this chance to present myself. All the male applicants wore navy blue suits with red power ties, as did many of the women. Things were going extremely well—that is, until my last of four interviews.

Despite being a biology major, I'd had the opportunity and was encouraged to take a number of elective classes in addition to my foreign language requirement. In high school I had taken French, which I wanted nothing to do with in college, so I decided to study Hebrew. I grew up in a fairly religious home, and my grandparents were Orthodox, which means they were very strict with the rules. I had lived with all the rituals but was short on explanations, so by the time I went to college, I wanted to know more about my own traditions as well as those of other religions. As a result, I took a fair number of comparative religion classes, which I found fascinating and a great diversion from the hard-core premed requirements. We studied the Torah and the New Testament and compared them with other religions of the world. I was able to converse fairly well in Hebrew after two years of almost one-on-one instruction in a small class taught by an attractive twenty-four-year-old Israeli woman. Because most of the guys were enamored of her, we studied extra to impress her.

My last interview at the medical school was with a full professor who specialized in internal medicine. He looked at my transcript and took note of the religion classes in particular. "In looking at your record, Bruce, I think that you should become a rabbi."

"Thank you, I guess." He wasn't Jewish.

He continued to press me on my decision to take so many religion classes and asked again why I wanted to be a physician. Not satisfied with my answers, he insisted that I should go on to rabbinic training. I calmly responded for the third time by reciting my well-rehearsed statement about why I wanted to be a physician. Once again, and this time more vehemently, he pushed me away from medicine and toward becoming a rabbi, seemingly annoyed with our entire discussion.

I don't know if this interviewer was having a bad day, didn't like me or my application, or just didn't like Jews. (Or maybe he thought the world needed more rabbis!) Either way, the interview went from bad to worse, and I left feeling completely deflated, knowing

I was not going to be admitted to the school where my chances were the highest. I found his questions neither pertinent nor appropriate, but I had no idea what to do. At my parents' urging, I called the admissions department to see if I could arrange another interview. They said they would consider my request, but another opportunity never materialized. Needless to say, I didn't get accepted to that school or any other that year.

Based on my classmates' experiences in Illinois, it was obvious to me that there were far fewer positions available in my home state, and this experience may have knocked me out of contention altogether. It bothered me that my premed classmates who were Illinois residents and had graduated with lower grade point averages than mine had already been accepted to medical schools. There were simply more slots available in Illinois for the number of students applying. I realized that my best option at that point was to change my residence and apply again. Actually, it wasn't a bad idea, since this meant living in Chicago for the year and growing up even more.

* * *

I didn't have a problem finding a job related to biology or medicine. There was a research assistant position listed at Michael Reese Hospital on the south side, affiliated with the University of Chicago. The annual salary was $15,000, which I thought was a terrific sum of money. I unrealistically figured that with that kind of cash (calculated at $7.81 an hour), I could send my grandparents on a well-deserved vacation, buy gifts for my friends and family, and do some traveling. After a day of searching, I was able to find an apartment in downtown Chicago that was affordable, situated over a hair salon in what was known as a transition neighborhood. This meant that when you walked out the front door, you'd better turn right and never left, especially after dark. Walk quickly, keep your head down, and avoid eye contact with anyone who passed you. In reality, I wasn't afraid. I felt confident that I knew how to keep myself out of trouble in most urban settings by this time.

Work was intense yet interesting. I was employed by a group that did research on kidney stone disease. Our studies were basic, performed on cells or blood samples from laboratory rats. Each week, all twenty of us, both investigators and assistants, assembled to review what we had accomplished over the preceding five days.

"Show me the data," the chairman demanded. "How can you not have new data from a whole week's worth of work?" There was a lot of pressure to produce results and have them analyzed on the only available computer in time for the meeting. This state-of-the-art computer system was housed in a frigid room the size of a small McDonald's franchise. Every Friday, the research assistants entered their results for the week and attempted to have some progress to report.

My hours were well over the forty per week I was being paid for. I often came in on weekends to care for and assess the animals used in our studies. I justified the extra hours with my supervising physician's promise that I would be named as a coauthor on the final paper. I was also getting excellent letters of recommendation for my medical school application.

Life was pretty simple. I was twenty-two years old, still involved in academics, and getting paid for it. I enjoyed my off-hours and living in the heart of the city. I was now part of the real world, waiting to get into medical school, but I wasn't ready to let go of basketball. I joined a downtown YMCA and played in nightly pickup games with an assortment of city characters. Basketball kept me calm as it had my entire life, and it also kept me in shape. The Y was a welcome contrast to my daytime world populated by University of Chicago professors, and it served as a much-needed distraction.

I applied once again to medical school, this time as an Illinois resident, and was accepted to a few schools. I chose to attend the Medical College of Virginia. The basic research on kidney stone disease would prove to be an invaluable experience and undoubtedly contributed to my eventual decision to become a urologist. My only disappointment was that I was never listed as a coauthor of the published paper, despite the repeated promises throughout my days and weekends of extended hours. I didn't learn of the decision until midway through my first year at medical school when I received a call from my supervising physician, who blamed the decision on the chairman and gave no other explanation. I was surprised that he didn't stand up for me since he'd witnessed how hard I'd worked. It hurt to have been deceived, but it didn't knock me down too far. I simply decided to take this as an important lesson on how not to treat those at a lower rank in training or status when I reached a position of power or influence.

After a day or two, I didn't give the episode a second thought. After all, I was in medical school and had a whole lot on my plate. It was great to finally be in this position and starting to move closer to reaching my goal of becoming a doctor.

Chapter Ten:

EXIT MEDICAL SCHOOL A DIFFERENT PERSON

High school is supposed to get you ready for college, which was not true in my case, so I couldn't help but wonder if college had prepared me for medical school. It turned out that Northwestern had, at least from an academic standpoint. However, nothing can ever truly prepare you emotionally to become a physician.

At the Medical College of Virginia, we began our studies forewarned we'd be learning at a pace five times that of the average college class. It sounded intimidating when we arrived, but once we got down to the work, it was fine. We knew that we were studying for a purpose and were ready to embark on our chosen profession. Our classes began at eight in the morning, and with only an hour for lunch, we sat through seven or eight lectures every day.

At the beginning of each week, we would receive a syllabus for the next five days of lectures. Usually the notes were complete, but some professors would supply only an outline and expect you to fill in the information as they lectured. Classes then consisted of taking exact notes as the instructor spoke. We were responsible not only for every word printed on those pages but also any statement uttered in class. Some lectures were entertaining and witty, while others were focused and inspiring. Still, it wasn't uncommon to fall asleep in class, especially when the lights were dimmed or after lunch as the information was delivered in a monotone. You just hoped you didn't breathe too loudly.

Missing a class or not picking up every point was usually not a problem since medical students were more than happy to help each other out. You could always obtain a copy of someone else's notes or go over what you missed after class. We constantly repeated our mantra, P = MD, meaning all you had to do was pass (P) in order to graduate and become a medical (M) doctor (D). Most of us did much better than a passing grade, but we still never refused to assist a classmate due to competition. It was very different from our college experience, and with the hordes of information we were responsible for, this camaraderie helped keep the pressure manageable.

The first two years of medical school taught all of us how far our minds could be pushed and challenged. Our weekly handouts usually ran more than five hundred pages. Rarely did we have the luxury of reading them more than once, and never more than twice, before we were tested on the material. I believe the ability to overcome these rigorous academic challenges is important in giving physicians the confidence necessary to understand how far they can be pushed and how successful they can be as a result.

In my case, having grown up with such profound self-doubt regarding my own intellect due to all the athlete stereotyping, it was even more important. After graduating from medical school, I would never again have those concerns. It was a good feeling.

As we moved further along in medical school and were pressed further to excel, our growth increased at an overwhelming rate. But often it had little to do with our studies. At the start of our first year, the upper-level medical students levied two stern warnings. The first was not to fall into the trap of studying twenty-four hours a day, seven days a week because even if you did, you still would not believe you knew the material well enough. The second warning was related to the first: to not spend all your time studying. "After all," they told us, "you'll only be in your twenties once!"

Within the first few months, after we found our bearings and got into a routine, my buddies and I took these recommendations to heart. We worked hard, but we played hard as well. Our social lives were important to us, as were athletics. It was then that basketball returned to my life, stronger than ever.

Had I known how prominent and important the school's gym was to so many of the students and faculty members, I never would have applied anywhere else. During our first two years, our classroom instruction was completed by 3:00 or 4:00 p.m., and shortly thereafter we met at the gym, whose two regulation full courts were almost always filled. Medical, dental, nursing, physical therapy, and graduate students as well as professors and physicians all had complete access. There was a well-used weight room to the side of the gym, but the basketball court was the main attraction, and it's probably where I played at the highest level of my life.

Despite our academic obligations, ten or more guys from my class somehow managed to get in two or three hours of basketball a day. We had a lot of steam to blow off. We were young and had just sat through eight hours of lectures, and basketball allowed us to keep our sanity. The competition on the court was incredible. Many of the guys who showed up daily had played college ball, and quite a few regulars had played in the ACC at places like the University of North Carolina and the University of Virginia. Many others came from competitive smaller schools in the area, such as James Madison University, George Mason University, and Hampton University. I learned early on that I would rather study three hours in a fit, well-rested state than study six hours mentally fatigued. It seemed like common sense to me, but not everyone understood or agreed with my philosophy. Basketball again grounded me, kept me focused, and let me clear my head for a few hours each day.

Intramural games were important, and each class from all the schools had at least one team. During our second year, our team went on to win the championship for the league, which was competitive and highly prestigious. As a prize, we were given T–shirts proclaiming our status, which we wore proudly. In addition, at the end of the season, one player came up with the idea of putting together an all-star team that challenged a similar squad from the undergraduate college, Virginia Commonwealth University. The game took place at the Richmond Coliseum, and I was asked to be a part of the team of twelve. Despite our opponents being a few years younger than us, we destroyed them. After all, our graduate team was dominated by former collegiate athletes, whereas, by definition, the undergraduate team had none. The VCU varsity squad, on the other hand, would have beaten us badly if they had been allowed to play in a pickup game like this. Regardless, the exciting, high-level game was a fitting sendoff after two years of hard study. Playing ball over the next few years, when I was in clinical rotations, would prove more difficult.

As our third year of medical training began, time was no longer spent in the classroom but in hospital wards, and our hours were much less predictable. As I discovered what it really meant to be a physician, basketball played a minor role in my life.

How do you teach a medical student about being responsible for another person's life? How does he or she learn about mortality? As my classmates and I began our third year, we were all quickly confronted with complicated issues. Sure, many of us had complex life experiences already, but rarely of the intensity and frequency that we were exposed to in the next phase of our training. More important than anything, we needed experience in understanding our own responses to a critical mistake or a less-than-ideal judgment in patient care. In such cases, not only would the patient do poorly, but in retrospect, you would see that your own action or inaction may have contributed to the outcome. Where does one learn to cope with the guilt and the resulting self-doubt? The answer was this was never taught, and it wasn't easy to figure out on your own .

For the first two years of medical school, the illnesses and the diseases we studied were abstract, read about only in books, viewed on an X-ray screen, or seen under a microscope. Third year, however, attached a name, a face, and a family to the disease process, and I believe that is what changed us forever. As third-year students, we not only learned the practice of medicine through discussions and readings, but we received a great deal of on-the-job training. We were given immense responsibilities as we entered our clinical rotations, and there was no room for, or acceptance of, miscalculations. We were expected to learn under fire.

"See one, do one, teach one" was the doctrine that medical students and residents had lived by for one hundred years. Yet in our experience, I'm not sure we always "saw one" first.

With my rotation on the general surgical service, I was introduced to a poor, inebriated man who had been involved in an altercation and was beaten up badly. His face had been shattered by being hit with a toilet seat cover. This incident involving an interesting choice of weapon was only one of the many stories we heard working in the emergency room over the years. The intern I was working with at the time, a guy two years ahead of me in training and whom I knew well from our years on the basketball court, told me the patient had already been assessed and cleared for any neurological injuries. Now his main problems were the numerous skin lacerations over his face and head.

"Hey, Bruce," he said, "your turn to work here. I need you to sew him up and make this look like a face again."

"Great," I said. "Only one problem: I've never sutured before."

"No sweat, I learned the same way. Just use an instrument tie," he told me, referring to the common suture technique. "Look, I'll show you." He pulled an orange from his lab-coat pocket, did a quick stitch or two, and shoved the orange into my hands. "Now you try." I fumbled through a couple stitches and began to get the hang of it. "Looks pretty good," the intern said. "Call me when you're done."

I had no idea what I was doing, but I eventually put more than two hundred sutures into the man's face, at first using Novocain around the open flesh but then realizing it wasn't necessary due to the alcohol-and-drug-induced coma. I carefully tied my sutures with perfect knots, despite the putrid smell of his breath and the head motion that accompanied each loud snore. Several hours later, task completed, I thought I'd done a pretty decent job, and I paged my intern to have him come and look at my handiwork. By then he had seen a number of critically ill patients elsewhere in the hospital.

"I'm sure it's fine, Bruce," he said over the phone. "Now get up here on the floor. We need to get a guy here ready for the OR. He may have a perforated bowel."

On the surgery rotation, approval often had to come from within. You needed to be mentally tough, and that may be why it eventually appealed to me as a specialty. Surgical service taught us about life and death because everything happened quickly. One minute you're talking to your patient and trying to calm him down, assuring him that everything is going to be fine, and the next moment he may die in front of you of massive injuries, all the time keeping eye contact and pleading with you to save his life. It was hard, and as medical students, we were never given any instruction on how to cope. We understood that while on the surgery rotation, there just wasn't time to look back. You needed to move on to the next crisis, and it always came quickly. The surgical service was challenging and pushed you to your limits, intellectually, physically, and emotionally, but it was on the general medical service that students had even more autonomy and more responsibility.

The majority of patients at MCV were indigent, poorly educated, uninsured, extremely nice, and usually very grateful for your help. The medical service was run by the senior resident, who was three to four years ahead of us in training but not a fully certified doctor yet. The attending physicians, who had the ultimate responsibility, would see the patients on rounds maybe once a week. For the most part, it was simply a formality since they rarely made a decision on cases or even heard about the outcomes. Medical students and residents were overwhelmed by the volume of patients we were expected to care for daily and the amount of effort it took.

At MCV, medical students were expected to draw all the blood before the day began, round on the patients twice a day, transport patients to radiology or anywhere else they needed to go, and do whatever was necessary to further the care of patients in a timely manner. The mindless jobs we were assigned were called "scut work," and it was never-ending. The tedious tasks relegated to medical students kept us in the hospital until late at night, and we'd have to return early in the morning to be certain that our patients were well cared for.

It seems ironic that we were the ones paying tuition to become educated, yet we were also expected to perform all the hospital work that was left undone. Those ahead of us in training called us "scut monkeys," but by spending so much time at the bedside, we became the patients' doctors in every sense of the word. That experience introduced us to having patients depend on our individual knowledge and skills. We began to feel the exhilaration that comes from helping someone and making a difference, but also the weight of the responsibility.

Name tags were given to us on the first day of medical school for us to wear until we graduated. Mine said "BA Rosenfeld" and below that, "M86," meaning I was in medical school and was scheduled to graduate in 1986. After a rough night of multiple admissions, no sleep, and preparation for a case presentation on the medical service, our group of residents and medical students performed 5:30 a.m. walk rounds. That was when we saw the patients on our service and went over the plans for the day.

I had been caring for a Mr. Harold Jackson, an emaciated, seventy-two-year-old admitted for dehydration, urinary tract infection, newly diagnosed heart disease, and renal insufficiency. After I'd spent three days monitoring his vital signs and labs, adjusting his medication, and giving him intravenous fluids, he was ready to go home. During his hospitalization, I had become quite fond of Mr. Jackson, getting to know him well and learning all about his life and family. Whether I was drawing his blood or taking him to X-ray, I was the only person from our service he saw regularly. I wanted to do everything perfectly; I tried to be compassionate and worked hard to treat his ailments. On this day he felt better than he had in years and looked forward to keeping up with his health.

While we were on rounds, the senior resident asked Mr. Jackson the name of his doctor, whom he would follow up with to be certain his condition didn't relapse or worsen. He smiled a wide, toothless grin and proudly exclaimed, "My doctor is B. A. Rosenfled." We all laughed and commented on his enthusiasm. I got kidded about this for weeks and now had a new nickname, but I was happy that at least for this hospitalization, I really had been his doctor and had done a great job. Because of my efforts, Mr. Jackson was in much better condition than he had been in a long time. I was now learning just why I'd entered the profession in the first place.

* * *

From day one of medical school, our professors promised that by the time we graduated, we would become completely different people. That prediction proved to be absolutely correct. The most profound metamorphosis occurred during our third year. For the first time, we participated directly in matters of life and death while working at the hospital. Whether it was discussing a new terminal diagnosis outside the room of a patient about to be informed of their fate or witnessing a body slowly being eaten away by a vengeful cancer, it made even a cocky, self-absorbed twenty-four-year-old grow up pretty quickly. Talking to a man with lung cancer and watching his minor coughing turn into a pulmonary artery erosion with liters of blood lost in a matter of seconds is profound. You never forget the look of confusion, pleading, and despair on the patient's face as you watch the life drain out while you frantically try to avert the inevitable, knowing there's no chance you'll be successful. You could not avoid being affected by the trauma resuscitations and the numerous deaths we tried to deflect. Stabbing and shooting mortalities were somehow less bothersome, since in most cases you could console yourself by considering that these individuals had simply been on the receiving end of the same carnage they'd inflicted on someone else.

We entered medical school young, immature, and often brazen. We were constantly reminded that we were the "best and the brightest," and we believed that the world owed us everything we desired. Then came the change, as if on cue. We got serious because we finally understood exactly what stakes we were playing for. Medical school was fun and exciting but certainly not fun and games. We quickly learned that real people depended on us, and unfortunately, the graduating class of 1986 at the Medical College of Virginia learned this lesson of mortality on an even more personal level.

After graduating from the University of Notre Dame, Tim Collins started medical school in 1982, ready to take on the world. He was a black kid from Virginia Beach and the first in his family to go to college, let alone medical school. I knew him well because we played a lot of basketball together over the first two years. He was a solid guy, somewhere around 6'3", and had incredible natural ability. Rumor had it that Digger Phelps, Notre Dame's legendary basketball coach, had requested that Tim try out for the Irish but that he declined. More than once, I told Tim that if I had had half his innate talent, I wouldn't be in medical school but in the NBA. He'd just laugh and say, "Bruce, you say that, but you know you wouldn't." Truly, I guarantee that I would have.

Tim was a bright student and very popular with his classmates and professors. He wasn't afraid of hard work, and during one of our rotations together at the start of our third year, we managed to have a great time while taking excellent care of our patients, despite the long hours. We all greatly admired his cool and positive demeanor. He was already an excellent clinician, practicing with a high level of compassion while maintaining a sense of humor and professionalism. With the odds very much against him, Tim had made a lot of good choices along the way, and it was easy to see that he was going to be an incredible pediatrician, his chosen field.

Two months before graduation, after stopping to go into a drugstore in downtown Richmond, Tim was carjacked and shot, execution-style, by his assailants. The news was surreal; our graduating class was devastated.

I barely remember graduation day except that Tim's mom accepted the diploma for her son. He was one of those people destined for greatness, someone who would change the world, and the opportunity had been senselessly denied. All of us sobbed through the ceremony; in fact, I don't even recall taking the Hippocratic Oath. I know we must have, but I certainly can't remember it.

Just as our instructors had predicted, in four short years, we were all very changed people. We had laughed, cried, and grown up together. Now it was time to move on; our lives would never be the same. There was no doubt that we were all serious about our chosen profession and ready to be real doctors.

Chapter Eleven:

THE EARLY YEARS OF AIDS

I was accepted by the State University of New York at Buffalo for my first two years in general surgery, to be followed by three years in urology. To those not familiar, urology might seem a strange choice of specialty, but my decision was simple. Most medical students first choose between surgery and medicine, usually based on personality, bias, and probably most important, experience in the medical school rotation. I chose urology because I wanted to be a surgeon and because the field offered a great variety of options. You could treat men, women, and children. You could specialize in large cancer surgeries, smaller technical procedures, or both. Plus, I seemed to get along well with those I'd met in the field.

I was happy with my choice of specialty and lucky to have been accepted into a highly competitive surgical field. However, at this time, there was an emerging disease process that made cutting into patients a lot riskier than it had ever been in the past; this was the beginning of our experience with the AIDS virus.

As students, we'd first heard of this rare, nondescript virus two years before, in 1984. Back in our second year of medical school, the most difficult course, due to the excessive amount of memorization required, was Immunology and Infection. We studied bacteria, viruses, and the immune system, but throughout the entire four-week course, only one paragraph was allocated to the description of AIDS. The virus was called HTLV-3, and we were told that it was seen only in select populations, referred to as the five H's: homosexuals, heroin addicts, hemophiliacs, Haitians, and (w)hores. It was not yet known how this disease decimated the immune system or how it was transmitted, but it wasn't a major concern, since it only affected such relatively small and specific populations.

At the time, some very bright MCV instructors still believed this disease's impact on society would be inconsequential, that it was simply part of the throngs of minutiae we should know for exams yet held little clinical relevance.

The next year and during my third-year pediatric rotation, we were surprised to find a patient with the disease on our service. Baby Tashika was a four-month-old girl when I met her. She'd been born to a sixteen-year-old mother, an IV-drug user and prostitute, who died shortly after childbirth of overwhelming infection due to HTLV-3. Since Tashika had acquired the virus from her mother, she also suffered from severe infections and had been fighting for her life for months throughout her short existence in the hospital. With her mother gone and no other family member interested, this baby's entire socialization came from her interactions with the caring nurses and doctors in training who worked so hard to keep her alive. Nobody realized or was willing to admit that her chance of long-term survival was essentially zero.

As third-year medical students, we were eager to do anything necessary to help this adorable, joyful child even though her needs took up much of our time and resources. Intravenous access was almost always a problem for patients this age and especially those so ill, and when a new IV line was necessary, the first attempts were often left to the medical student. We all knew about her diagnosis and the virus that had caused her illness, but we were not concerned for our own safety since we had been told repeatedly we were not at risk of transmission. She was often cared for and treated without any basic personal protection such as gloves, face masks, gowns, or eye covers. We were assured continuously by the attending physicians that no healthcare worker had ever caught this virus through patient contact. It was thought that the amount of virus needed to contract this disease was so high that one could never become infected with something as minimal as a needle stick or a spurt of blood to the eye.

Even that early in my career, that logic made no sense to me. We all knew that this child had a horrible disease she'd contracted from her mother, who herself had been infected by another. It just didn't seem right that healthcare providers could afford to be cavalier with her contaminated blood. We didn't think that way about hepatitis; why was this infectious disease so different? I personally witnessed countless medical students and residents get stuck with this baby's contaminated needles because they were working so quickly, and nobody was concerned about the implications of a stick. One code blue stands out in particular.

One day Tashika couldn't breathe. As residents worked once again to prolong this baby's life, blood began flying everywhere. Counter to the norm, I walked around in gloves and other protective gear, picking up the multitude of contaminated needles strewn over the bed and surrounding area and placing them in a sharps container to prevent any accidents. The same scene was repeated numerous times until, a few weeks later, Tashika finally died. We were saddened when she couldn't be revived a final time but took comfort knowing that at least the poor child was finally out of pain.

The casual attitude toward this disease didn't last much longer. By the end of my fourth year as I was about to start my general surgery residency, the medical profession had gained a greater understanding of the newly named AIDS virus and its mode of transmission. Reports started coming out that described nurses and doctors dying from this virus transmitted through needle sticks and common hospital procedures. Now everyone involved with care of this disease was petrified, and the hospitals went to the other extreme in dealing with these patients. Suddenly, most providers couldn't stay far enough away from these patients. Upon being diagnosed with HIV or AIDS, the patient was placed in an isolation room with minimum contact recommended. If these poor people left their rooms, they were expected to wear a gown and a mask. The staff usually wore the same, and in some hospitals, it looked like we were wearing space suits just to speak with the patients. I didn't buy into this extreme either since discharged patients were given no special instructions regarding interaction with their families or the general public. How could contact be so risky in the hospital and then of no concern on the street? Nothing we were doing seemed to make sense, but we continued taking extreme measures because we were so afraid of contracting the virus. This was especially true among surgeons, since most HIV or

AIDS patients required a surgical procedure to be diagnosed.

In the early years of AIDS, patients often presented with enlarged lymph nodes. To make a diagnosis, one of the nodes would be excised and analyzed under a microscope. Since fear was rampant even among the attending doctors, the procedure was often assigned to the lowest-ranking surgeon on the service, the intern who was less than a year out of medical school. This was also the least experienced person and hence the most likely to stick themselves or others with a scalpel or a needle. It wasn't fair or appropriate, but the attending physicians didn't mind shirking this high-risk responsibility. Luckily, this scenario lasted only about a year, when a blood test became available.

In a surgery residency, needle sticks were often unavoidable, something we dreaded but viewed as an acceptable risk, at least before AIDS came along. Eventually, the risk was minimized as we became accustomed to universal precautions, which meant treating every patient as if he or she had full-blown AIDS and being extremely careful at all times. For us to survive, our culture as physicians and surgeons had to change.

Upon completing medical school and residency training, I was required to get an HIV screening in order to buy life insurance. This would be my first test after having experienced so many mishaps standard for medical students and surgical residents over the past seven years. I was on edge until I received the negative results. It's all second nature now, but we understood that to survive, we had to quickly learn how to protect ourselves.

Chapter Twelve:

REMEMBER, CALLING IS A SIGN OF WEAKNESS

Urology is considered a surgical subspecialty, and to start that residency program, I would have to get through the prerequisite two years of general surgery training. It was such a difficult task that at one point, my medical school classmates informed me they had a betting pool and that the odds of my successfully completing two years of general surgery weren't good. They thought that I was just too nice to adapt to the often cutthroat culture general surgery was known for.

I arrived in Buffalo at the end of June 1986 and joined a high-caliber bunch of newly graduated

medical doctors to begin our general surgery internship and then residency training. The group included
those who would stay in this program to become
general surgeons as well as those slated to go on to
other surgical subspecialties, such as otolaryngol-
ogy, orthopedics, plastic surgery, cardiac surgery, and
urology. On our first day, we received beepers, name
tags, and three pairs of white intern's pants to wear
with our long white coats. My beginning rotation was
the surgical intensive care unit at the Veterans Hospital, where you were responsible for ten to twenty
critically ill patients at any one time. In the mornings,
we would round with the attending physicians and go
over the plans and goals for the patients for that day.
The surgical ICU was a great place to start since the
patients' conditions were complex; you learned how
to organize and categorize a problem list to cover all
aspects of their illness. The days were busy, but there
were usually plenty of people around to ask questions
if there was ever a problem. As fresh MDs, the work-
load didn't bother us. And even though the learning
curve was steep, we pushed ourselves to understand
quickly, knowing this would be essential when we

needed to make independent decisions. This turned out to be sooner than we would have liked—on day one, actually.

"Feel free to call me if you have any problems at all," the senior resident told us on our first night as he was about to go home on backup call. Then he half-heartedly stated, "But remember, calling is a sign of weakness." As interns, we took his words as a warning, not a joke. From our first day, we were expected to run the surgical service during the night and call for assistance only in dire circumstances. With two surgical interns covering the entire hospital, we relied heavily on one another.

During my evenings on call, I covered the surgical ICU, and my co-intern covered the emergency room and surgical wards. Any problems, concerns, or management issues were ours to deal with. Any procedures, such as intubations or placement of catheters, central lines, or chest tubes, were for us to perform. The nights were hectic due to the complexity of patient problems as well as the tremendous amount of basic scut work to be completed before morning rounds. We didn't want to make a single mistake, and what we lacked in experience and knowledge we made up for in effort. The last thing we wanted was to face the scrutiny of a Monday-morning quarterback session by the surgical attending, second-guessing our decisions and questioning whether we had what it took to be a surgeon. Just one mistake could be grounds for dismissal from the program, and not having the proper training was no excuse.

One night my beeper screeched out instructions, calling me to a code blue on the ward. I was the first to arrive, and there were no anesthesiologists present. The poor man couldn't breathe; he was hypoxic and frantically trying to suck any available air into his lungs. Due to pneumonia and underlying lung disease, Mr. Baker had become unable to breathe on his own. Panic and pleading filled his eyes, and we both knew that he was very close to death.

The nursing staff pushed the code cart next to his bed, and since I was the only physician present, I knew that I had to intubate this man. I had seen this procedure performed many times and had tried once while being observed in the operating room, but I had never attempted it on my own. I wasn't confident in my skills, but I hoped my knowledge of the anatomy would get me through.

The nursing staff assisted me, being as supportive as possible given my lack of experience and the difficult position we were in. I quickly assessed the patient's airway by looking down his throat with a laryngo-scope and tried to determine exactly where to place the tube. He was attached to a cardiac monitor, and we knew that if we could not get the breathing tube in right away, he would be dead within minutes.

Mr. Baker began to vomit, which made seeing the throat structures even more difficult, and I was con-cerned that he would aspirate the fluid into his lungs, which in itself could be fatal. I failed to place the endotracheal tube on the first attempt, so I removed the tube, suctioned the area, and tried again, pray-ing that the tube went in the proper area. My second attempt was successful, and he was quickly attached to a mechanical ventilator by a nurse assisting. Sup-port then arrived from other interns on various ser-vices, and we all congratulated each other on "saving another." The patient was transported to the medical

ICU, and I didn't hear any follow up after that point. I was curious but had already moved on to the next crisis, so I didn't give the incident further consideration. There would be no feedback by my attending staff and no recognition for a job well done. I would have heard from my superiors only if the patient had not survived.

Several months later, a well-dressed man came up to me and said he had trouble tracking me down but wanted to shake my hand. He told me that he had graduated with a business degree from Northwestern long before I'd been there and that he knew he could always count on a fellow Wildcat when he needed assistance. I knew then that some higher power was helping me that night—or that something or someone was looking after Mr. Baker.

Chapter Thirteen:

MAYBE LAW SCHOOL IS MY FUTURE

Most people outside medicine don't understand the difference between an intern and a resident. Typically, the intern year is the first year of training after medical school and is pretty basic. Residents are any physicians in training programs who have finished their internships. As they move through the residency program, they are known first as junior residents, then senior residents, and finally chief residents. It's a little different now but basically the concept is the same. In my program, I was on call in the hospital every other night for two years straight, first as an intern in general surgery and then as a first-year resident. In both positions, being on call for surgery meant you were in the hospital, providing direct patient care and carrying a pager so you could be available within minutes for any emergency. The time commitment of this tradition was incomprehensible.

Here's what a typical week looked like. We would arrive at the hospital on a Monday at 5:00 a.m. We assisted in blood draws and morning rounds on patients and ensured those scheduled for the operating room were prepared. If we were lucky, we might have time to grab a quick breakfast. During the day, our responsibilities included seeing patients in the outpatient clinic, assisting with surgical cases, and performing any task required to make the service run smoothly, such as checking test results or starting IVs. If we were fortunate, we repeated patient rounds in the late afternoon instead of the early evening. The rounds took as long as was necessary to see the patients on our service and assign tasks for their care. The lowest ranking on the service then completed the generated scut work.

Nighttime coverage usually overwhelmed us due to the huge responsibility and significant understaffing, but it also taught us the importance of triage. This meant completing the serious tasks first and leaving those less pressing for later. If you got any sleep while on call, it was usually less than three or four hours with many interruptions.

The next day started again at 5:00 a.m. as we were joined by our fellow residents fortunate enough to have spent a few hours sleeping at home. Tuesday would proceed as Monday had, and if we were lucky, we would get home by 7:00 p.m. Keep in mind that we had arrived at five in the morning the day before and had been working for thirty-eight hours straight. We barely made it home and immediately fell asleep before it was time to get back to the hospital at five o'clock Wednesday morning. We resisted adding up our hours at the time, but it typically ended up being about a 133-hour workweek. The same brutal schedule continued for two straight years, and being fatigued was never an acceptable excuse for making a less than perfect decision. Despite these long hours, we were paid by the state of New York for only 37.5 hours— not even the standard 40. The state thought that we shouldn't be compensated for our thirty-minute lunch breaks.

Despite being a licensed physician with extensive responsibilities, I was compensated as a first-year intern at $4.31 an hour. However, it seemed like a fantastic sum of money at the time. Having been a perpetual student up to that point, I was thrilled to have a little cash to spend, even if there was no time to do so. Thank goodness my student loans remained deferred despite their compounding a ton of interest, or I wouldn't have been able to survive. At that time, we just didn't worry about the low pay, the absurd hours, and the obviously unfair nature of the entire arrangement. We had one purpose: to develop surgical skills and become exceptional physicians and surgeons. We did whatever it took to achieve that goal, and mostly without complaint. Complaining was considered a sign of weakness, and as a surgeon, that was the last trait you wanted to exhibit.

At SUNY Buffalo, we cared for the state's prisoners, the homeless, and the drug-addicted. We cared for people who were infected with HIV or had full-blown AIDS and anyone with any disease at any time. Mostly we treated patients who were shunned by society, couldn't pay for care, or both. In dealing with this group, I felt fortunate to have grown up on the playground since it exposed me to people of all backgrounds and taught me to relate to all people. As a result, I didn't feel out of touch with my patients.

As an intern, if you weren't working, you were expected to be studying. In our program, the conferences were where we learned the most. These conferences were held frequently and presented by interns, residents, and attending doctors. There might be a pre-op conference, where we discussed patients who were going on to surgery, as well as pediatric and oncology conferences. Grand Rounds and Morbidity & Mortality conferences both were important opportunities for learning. Grand Rounds was an hour presentation, usually given by a resident on a disease or technique, describing cases for review with professional slides of X-rays and pathology. The talks often took weeks to put together, were well attended, and gave residents an opportunity to shine. The most interesting conference, however, and certainly the most entertaining, was the Morbidity & Mortality conference. Blood was often spilled, and you never knew if residents might be fired or reprimanded for their actions.

M&M was usually held once a week, and attendance was mandatory for interns, residents, and even attending physicians. The chairman of general surgery always led the conference and worked from a list of cases the residents were required to present. The presentations concerned patients who had experienced adverse outcomes and had either died or suffered complications of one sort or another. If an intern or a resident were involved with a particular case in any way, they were expected to know every detail and understand fully the controversial judgment that may have occurred. They also had to be able to present and describe the pertinent literature to both support and refute the position on how it would have been handled best. The conference was frequently traumatic to those presenting, and its purpose was to allow doctors in training to defend their actions and teach their colleagues a better way to handle similar cases in the future.

In this high-stress forum, the most important rule when presenting was never to talk about anything you weren't completely certain of. You couldn't ever make up a story or fill in the blanks since the chairman had studied the cases and knew more about them than you did, and certainly more about disease process and its proper treatment. Also, you could never be afraid to say the three magic words—"I don't know"—or admit you might have acted differently with the benefit of hindsight. If you did, the conversation then commonly would veer off in another direction, and the chopping block was set aside for another day or another victim.

I once witnessed a senior resident in general surgery (meaning a thirty-two-year-old physician in his fourth year out of five in his surgical training) give a poorly informed response when queried on the hospital course of a specific patient. It was obvious from his answers that his familiarity with the case and understanding of the disease process were not where they should have been. Our chairman used this opportunity to pronounce judgment in front of the entire surgical program. "It's obvious that there's a problem with your knowledge base, but certainly nothing that repeating a full year of training won't correct."

The resident staff learned very early that M&M was something to be feared, and the best possible scenario was to remain as invisible as possible. As intimidating as it was, so long as you weren't the one being hammered, it was also a tremendous learning experience.

In January of my first year of residency, I was about to begin my second rotation through the surgical ICU, this time at a private hospital where the instruction was reportedly more intense. Theoretically, that was good since there was a potential for greater learning, but there was only one minor concern. From what I'd heard, the attending who ran the ICU believed residents were best taught by designating one as incompetent at the beginning of the three-month rotation and then constantly pointing out this individual's shortcomings. Life was fine as long as you weren't the chosen one, and I wasn't concerned the attending would bestow that honor on me. After all, I had never been bullied my entire life, and I was sure it wasn't about to start now.

There were three surgery residents and one anesthesiology resident in this rotation, and we were all good team players. It was far enough into the year that we were starting to gain confidence in our knowledge and our skills. During the first week of the rotation, the attending seemed competent and encouraging and didn't really bother any of us. I began to suspect that the rumors about his teaching methodology had been fabricated as a scare tactic. The following week, however, everything changed.

"Bruce, why did you give that patient half normal saline and not the Ringer's lactate that I specifically wanted?" "Bruce, why isn't that IV working? Can't you place a simple line correctly?" Obviously, I had been designated the idiot of the rotation. My patients were doing well, and I hadn't made any real mistakes that any of us were aware of. I was to be the scapegoat for teaching purposes and could expect a lot of unfair treatment and even outright abuse at times. I wasn't sure why I'd received that distinction, but after two weeks of being belittled and humiliated nonstop, I knew something had to change.

This ICU was not as large as the one at the VA hospital, but the patients were probably more acutely ill, and the pressure for an exceptional outcome seemed higher. Despite those expectations, nights were just as understaffed, and calling for backup was still construed as a sign of weakness. Three weeks into the rotation, on Saturday morning rounds with our attending in full-attack mode, I lost my composure. I'd been up for thirty hours straight and had successfully resuscitated several patients throughout the night without assistance. It was only after being chewed out for the minutest detail that I lost my cool for the first and only time in my career. Every instinct that I'd learned on the playground in Metuchen came back to me, and it wasn't good.

There had been three very ill patients in the ICU the previous evening, any of whom might not have survived the night. Despite having earned my medical degree only six months before, I was left as the sole physician in charge of the unit. I was terrified of making the wrong decision, like most interns and even upper-level residents would have been in the same situation. I was unable to lie down for even five minutes, rotating among the three sick patients' rooms, changing medications, pushing fluids, and keeping them alive. They had minimal chances of survival long term, but I was not about to let any of them die on my watch.

The next morning, when my team returned for rounds, I was proud of my efforts and accomplishments and related my war stories to my intern colleagues, who seemed impressed and congratulated me. My attending, however, had a far different reaction.

"Bruce, I see that this patient required two liters of fluid, and for one of those liters, you used normal saline. That's ridiculous. I wanted you to give albumin instead. Don't you ever listen to anything I tell you?"

I defended my actions for the first time. "Sir, the patient was coding and close to death at the time, and we grabbed whatever fluid was closest in this dire situation. I was at his bedside, it was an emergency, and the albumin was not available."

"Not good enough!"

In reality, I had dealt with each of these situations appropriately, but because I was the designated incompetent for the rotation, nothing I could do would be considered correct.

After rounds, my fellow residents showed me their support by assuring me that they would have done exactly the same thing during last night's rotations. They sympathized with me, knowing that I had to take this sort of unwarranted abuse, and commiserated that there was nothing any of us could do about it. I wasn't so sure about that.

I figured I actually had several options. First, I could hit the attending with a flurry of f-bombs in front of the group and staff and then tell him where he could shove his bottle of albumin. Not a terrible idea, but it wouldn't have helped me get anywhere except searching for another training program. The second option was to wait for him to leave the hospital, meet him by his car, and push him around a bit. That probably would have felt even better than telling him off but more than likely would have gotten me arrested and barred from practicing medicine ever. Not a great option. Third, I could have cried out loud, curled into a fetal position, and felt sorry for myself, but I was too angry and way past that point. Eventually, I realized the only real alternative was to discuss my concerns with this attending face-to-face.

After rounds were over, I walked into my attending's office, closed the door, and sat down. I calmly informed him that I didn't understand his teaching style and couldn't fathom what I had done to incur his wrath to the point where everything wrong was my fault and a tremendous opportunity for my colleagues to learn how to not practice medicine. I informed him that this arrangement was unacceptable, and that if this manner of instruction continued, I would have no other choice but to drop out of this residency program and leave medicine altogether. He looked at me dumbfounded.

I then went on to explain the following. Having thrown my MD degree out the window, I would apply and get accepted to law school, graduate to eventually specialize in medical malpractice, and from there, I would devote my high-power law practice to reviewing his cases and his cases only, since I knew I would make a fortune given the abhorrent level of care he delivered. I then left his office without further discussion, creating the illusion of a lack of concern about any possible repercussions. Inside, I was completely torn apart and had no idea what would happen. There was nothing left to do but wait for the fallout.

The ICU attending never acknowledged the conversation, but after that day, he was as kind as could be to me. For weeks, I wondered if I was going to be called into the chairman's office and instructed to leave the program, but I never was. Several days later, all angst was redirected away from me and toward the anesthesia intern. From that day on, and for the next two months, I was taught very well, learned a lot, and was no longer criticized unmercifully. That was left for my unfortunate colleague, who seemed to tolerate it much better than I did, and we never stopped supporting him.

For the next few years, and even when I had completed general surgery and moved on to urology, this same attending was overly congenial to me, going out of his way to say hello and engage in small talk. I think he was afraid of me. I certainly had no intention of ever attending law school, but I knew things had to change, and I did what was necessary to make that happen. When it comes to intimidation and being able to defend myself, once again: Thank you, Franklin School playground!

Chapter Fourteen:

THE TRUTH JUST DOESN'T MATTER

Our first-year rotations were heavily weighted toward gaining experience in the ICU and the emergency room, which helped me learn how to treat acutely ill patients early on. One routine evening around 7:00 p.m., an extremely complex postoperative neurosurgical spine case was brought to my area after over ten hours in the OR. Our team was just finishing evening rounds when I broke away to get this guy settled in. Despite the length of the procedure, the patient was stable and would require nothing other than active monitoring. The neurosurgery residents had written the orders for his care, but because the patient was technically on the ICU service, the orders required a cosignature from both me and the ICU attending.

This was a good night for me because I was leaving for home relatively early, somewhere around 8:30, and I was happy I wasn't required to return until 5:30 the next morning. I was really looking forward to sleeping in my own bed.

After I left for home, one of my fellow interns covered the spine patient, who reportedly had an uneventful night. In the morning, the on-call intern checked him out to me after he had been seen by the neurosurgery team, whose resident had written his orders for transfer to a standard surgical floor. Per protocol, both my attending and I again cosigned the orders. The patient was transported to the surgical floor in excellent condition, alert and oriented with no special complaints, never to be seen again by any of us in the ICU.

Months later, I heard that the patient had gone on to have a complicated postsurgical course, and ultimately his spinal condition worsened after surgery.

He never required further ICU care, but his stay in the hospital and rehabilitation center ended up lasting over three months. Apparently, he was very unhappy with his outcome, which I could certainly empathize with.

Almost a year after my brief and uneventful encounter with this man, I received a hand-delivered registered letter informing me that I was the subject of a medical malpractice lawsuit. I was ordered to give a deposition and warned that under the law, I was not allowed to discuss the case with anyone except my lawyers—and yes, I had better find myself an attorney to defend my egregious actions. I was devastated, feeling guilty and isolated without understanding why this case was brought against me or knowing what to expect next.

Within the next few days, I was contacted by the program's medical malpractice insurance carrier, which had assigned me a lawyer I would meet with in several weeks. I don't think I slept at all until then. I was convinced my career was over. At least that's what the charges said when I read them closely. I took it all very literally, although I had no idea what action the lawsuit was referring to.

My assigned attorney was reassuring, confident, and supportive. She let me know that the plaintiff's counsel was using the "shotgun approach," suing everyone and anyone who had even the remotest contact with this patient. Five attending physicians were named in the case, along with fifteen residents, as well as the hospital and at least two companies that manufactured some of the equipment used. The plaintiff also personally sued several of the medical equipment company's product representatives. When I asked about this strategy—as had the other residents involved—the lawyer told me that so many of the residents were included in the suit because the plaintiff did not want to miss anyone or any institution with "deep pockets," and we were covered by the state of New York. A copy of the entire patient record was supplied to me which I reviewed and highlighted carefully, paying special attention to any direct involvement I'd had in the patient's care. After objectively reviewing the six-hundred-page document, I concluded that there was nothing remotely inappropriate about the care I'd provided and that my involvement was minimal. I also critically reviewed the entire hospitalization for others who may have been at fault and couldn't find a single problem with anyone's actions. I concluded that this was a difficult and risky case for this patient, and they simply had not achieved the result he had hoped for. I also understood that this didn't matter; someone had to pay.

Several months later, I reported for my scheduled deposition. I had come directly from being on duty at the hospital and would need to return, so my attire consisted of white intern's pants and a lab coat, both permanently stained with recent and old blood, a frayed button-down shirt and tie, and a scratched Casio watch with a calculator for computing drug dosages for pediatric cases. My sneakers, usually also blood stained, were rinsed off to show respect. I also brought one of the disposable pens the hospital received from drug companies advertising their products, but I didn't end up using it.

* * *

When I walked in, I was instructed to sit at the large mahogany table surrounded by thickly cushioned leather chairs. There was a stark contrast between my appearance and that of the lawyers—they all wore fashionable, expensive suits and imported shoes, accompanied by gold-plated pens and elaborate leather briefcases. There must have been eight attorneys in the room representing all sides, as well as a single stenographer and at least one assistant for each lawyer. My assigned lawyer sat next to me and tried to keep me relaxed. As I waited nervously for the formal deposition to begin, I noted that most of these people seemed to know each other well. They laughed often and inquired about each other's families as if they had been in this situation many times. I wondered how much each of these individuals was being paid to be present for my hour of questioning. Add it all together and it probably equaled my yearly salary.

Once the proceedings began, the plaintiff's lawyer asked me the same questions over and over, to the point where it became exasperating. He lingered on my minimal contact with this case, yet he asked me about the cosigned orders at least ten times, trying to trip me up by phrasing the question a little differently with every pass. It didn't rattle me since I had nothing to hide, but it was irritating. It was also clear that my deposition was an attempt to spin the facts and make me contradict myself so the plaintiff's attorneys might have something to work with. I had no problem keeping up with the line of questioning, but I could easily imagine how simple and unfair it would be to manipulate a witness who was not so accustomed to dealing with pressure, or wasn't on the same intellectual footing.

The deposition went on for what seemed an eternity, but in reality, it took less than forty minutes. Two realities struck me as I walked away from that experience. First, the entire process was all a game. It didn't appear that anyone was trying to discover the truth; instead, everyone was looking to shape the story to suit his or her best interests. I don't imagine that's earth-shattering news, but it was disappointing to witness firsthand so early in my career. My second realization was that the truth really didn't matter. Anyone with a reasonable medical background could review the records as I had and conclude that there was no fault in this case. I certainly couldn't say the patient was not harmed by the surgery, but he did have a horrible problem to begin with, and it was a risky procedure. It was also very well documented that without the surgery, he could end up worse than he would have with the surgery.

The case was litigated for close to ten years before being settled. The attending surgeon who performed the postsurgical case was the first to be dropped after a year or two because he was so powerful in his specialty that the opposition could find no one who would testify against him. The insurance company eventually settled the case with no admission of guilt by anyone, and the patient died of an unrelated illness many years before the judgment.

I spent a lot of time worrying about the lawsuit's possible repercussions on my career. I had to report this event to every hospital and license that I applied for thereafter, despite knowing that I had done nothing wrong. It made me realize that if you were involved in a lawsuit in which your medical decisions might have been in any way questionable, dealing with the second thoughts and guilt could be devastating.

Compensation for real medical malpractice is certainly warranted, but this case lingered in the courts for almost a decade without legitimate merit. It was another piece of my innocence that I wish I could have kept just a little longer.

Chapter Fifteen:

NEVER REMOVE
THE SHACKLES

As surgery interns and residents, we rotated through a number of hospitals and often found ourselves in difficult situations without an attending surgeon present. This independence was never more pronounced than in the emergency room. Our rotation through the ER lasted for two months at a time, with twenty-four hours on and twenty-four hours off. The hours sound intense, but at only eighty-four hours a week, this was actually a low time commitment compared with our rotations on the surgical floors. By this point in the program, staying up for twenty-four hours straight was simple, so we regarded ER rotation as a holiday.

* * *

While covering the emergency department, we often received advanced notice from ambulance crews that a serious trauma or gunshot wound was on the way. The call would generate a series of pages, and the residents on service were expected to be on the scene within minutes. We understood that the most senior ranking resident present would be in charge and run the evaluation and treatment of whatever disaster appeared. It was unusual to see an attending physician around when a trauma arrived, probably because violence and accidents occurred mostly at night when the attendings were at home with their families.

With the first call from the ambulance, three or four residents would rush to the trauma room to await the impending catastrophe. Although we were only in our twenties for the most part, we were confident we could deal with whatever would burst through that door. The first goal upon the patient's arrival was to secure the airway, and the second was to access the bloodstream to administer fluids and medication. Arterial lines, central lines, catheters, and whatever else were placed as needed. I often volunteered to put in the chest tube if required, which I enjoyed doing for some reason. The procedure involves using a scalpel to incise the skin over a rib, inserting a finger into the pleural space, and passing a large-caliber tube to drain usually sizable quantities of blood, fluid, or even air from the space to ventilate the lungs. It could be brutal, but these were life-and-death situations in which seconds often made the difference.

No matter which hospital we were stationed at, we took all comers, employed universal precautions, and were responsible for making split-second decisions with the full understanding that the case might end up in conference, requiring us to defend our decisions in front of the entire department. We took our responsibilities seriously and never questioned how we were being trained. We were all well aware that each of us was only one decision away from being ordered to repeat a year of training or being asked to leave the program—or even losing our medical license. It put us under great pressure, but most of the time we were too busy to give it much thought.

Our residency program also had the honor of providing medical care for the Attica State Prison, which housed the scariest and most massive individuals I had ever come across. At the time, inmates had no restrictions on yard activities, and prisoners often spent most of their days lifting weights. Couple that with easy access to drugs and steroids, and the inmates appeared to have superhuman strength and muscle mass. Many had psychiatric illnesses, and we also were informed that the overwhelming majority were HIV-positive as well as infected with hepatitis.

The inmates would be led through the hospital corridors, and we called their walk the "Attica Shuffle," referring to the awkward way they walked while wearing shackles around their wrists, waists, and ankles. Even escorted by several armed guards, some inmates escaped while at the hospital. A fellow surgical resident was assaulted in an inmate's attempted escape from the ER, but fortunately, he wasn't badly injured. Most of the time when I covered the emergency room, I had no concern for my own safety, thanks to my friend Alex, one of the security guards at the hospital. He often reassured me, "Don't worry, Doc, I got your back." That's all I needed to hear.

Alex was years past his glory days playing high school football at a local Buffalo powerhouse, but at 6'1" and 265 pounds, he was still big, strong, and fearless. He was also heavily armed. I don't think he was allowed to carry weapons, but one day he revealed to me the knives and blades hidden all over his body. Alex often hung with us in the ER on slow nights, talking sports, reflecting on life, or helping us finish off our orders of pizza and wings. Even on busy evenings, he always checked in to make sure we were all right since several hard-core inmates might be present at any given time, usually requiring sutures for lacerations sustained during prison altercations. There were also other patients in the ER who were just as intimidating as those from Attica. Many of these guys were "between prison terms," and in some ways, they were scarier than the inmates since they could wait for you in the parking lot if they were not completely satisfied with your service.

Like a prison, the county hospital emergency room had its own rules that were important to adhere to in order to survive. Some were passed down from resident to resident, and others were devised on your own. These were those rules I lived by:

1. Always prescribe minimal narcotics. If you don't follow this guideline, every junkie in town will follow you from day to day and hospital to hospital. How they got the schedules I couldn't figure out, but it was probably an inside source.

2. Never remove chains or shackles when examining a prisoner. My newly discovered talent was the art of performing a complete physical examination with chains in place, and that included a prostate examination. It's amazing what a little fear can do for your creativity.

3. Never deal with mean, bad people without having Alex around. The reasons for this are obvious.

4. Always measure the length of any laceration you sew up.

The last rule wasn't meant to protect us from our patients but from our bosses. I learned this early from an ER attending.

"Bruce, you need to be certain that you measure every wound and document its size. This is crucial." He pulled out a small metric ruler and demonstrated. "Look, this is three centimeters, and this is five." I couldn't have cared less, and I think this was the only time this guy actually taught us.

The ER physician's job was to sign off on everything we had done over the past twenty-four hours. He usually read the resident's note and rarely asked for clarification before putting signature to paper. In addition to signing the encounter, he needed to bill the responsible party for the work that had been performed.

Despite the residents' making critical decisions without any attending input and physically completing all the work, the ER attending was more concerned if the length of a sutured wound wasn't documented to his liking. In most cases, I was the only resident in the ER and usually had patient charts piled up and more patients waiting to be seen. There were nights when we would spend countless hours sewing up lacerations, and the last thing I was concerned about was being accurate about their size. It didn't change how I handled the patient, and it didn't affect my salary or learning. Frankly, this minor detail didn't matter, yet it was an extremely high priority for my attending physician because that was how he got paid. And to survive my surgical residency, I needed to keep him happy.

It wasn't just in the ER where residents did the work for nonpresent attendings. The surgical service had numerous consults throughout the hospital being treated for wounds. Once a day, if assigned to this particular service, we would walk around the hospital, spending most our time at the rehab or nursing home units, assessing wounds and making recommendations for continued care. It was not uncommon to see twenty or more such patients in a day. Regardless, we provided excellent care while becoming adept at wound evaluation and treatment. Once a month, our attending would go around seeing all these patients and signing all our notes, up to thirty on one chart if they were seen daily. Twenty patients for thirty days, and let's assume they were reimbursed even a minimal thirty-five dollars for each encounter. That's six hundred patient visits, so you can do the math. It doesn't happen anymore, but these guys had it pretty good.

By the spring of 1988, I was on the verge of completing my first two years in general surgery training. I had gone through a further metamorphosis by dealing with daily pressures that pushed my limits both intellectually and emotionally. In addition, the physical demands and expectations were grueling yet strengthening despite chronic sleep deprivation. By age twenty-nine, I had truly learned about life and death, and on a number of occasions, I had directly influenced those outcomes. I learned that to be a successful surgeon, I needed a hard shell and couldn't afford to dwell on an undesirable outcome. There was way too much work to be done, and caring for our own emotional vulnerabilities was not a luxury we could allow ourselves. The paradigm was never directly verbalized but was regularly implied.

Our chairman in general surgery was an intimidating presence and an incredibly demanding person who made us better doctors. We were taught that as surgeons, not only were we expected to know how to operate, but we were also required to know medicine as well as or better than the medical doctors. We were never permitted to call a consult from another specialty for any problem. If, for example, a patient's diabetes needed more intensive monitoring, or if we were having trouble getting someone's blood pressure under control, or if a patient was experiencing chest pain, we were expected to handle it ourselves. We spent a lot of time with deathly ill patients and were both guided and pushed to manage all possible situations. We were taught to be confident and even a bit arrogant based on our command of the literature and intense training. We had to possess extreme self-assurance to make split-second decisions. I began to enjoy being a surgeon and realized it was easy to compare this experience to my earlier years on the court:

After putting on my uniform, I would sit in the locker room and feel a little nervous, wondering if my time spent on the playground had taught me enough to handle the ball against my opponent's high skill level and lightning quickness. Once on the court, I would fake right, drive left, whirl with my left hand, and pull up for a short jumper that hit only the net. I realized that despite my opponent's innate ability, he wasn't going to stop me. I was prepared to succeed and confident of the outcome.

And today:

After putting on my surgical scrubs, I sit in the locker room and feel a little nervous about the upcoming case. The patient being wheeled into the OR has an eighteen-centimeter hemorrhaging kidney that must be removed to stop the blood loss and to try to cure the cancer. I know this is going to be difficult, and I question whether my training has prepared me well enough to perform the procedure. Once I'm in the OR, the case goes routinely. I move quickly to isolate and then tie off the blood supply. The kidney is mobilized and beginning to come out nicely. I realize this case isn't that difficult. I was prepared to succeed and confident of the outcome.

I can't say I enjoyed my two years as a resident in general surgery, but they did serve their purpose. By July 1988, I had beaten the odds and survived my surgical training program, contrary to the predictions of my medical school classmates. They all knew I had a passion for basketball, but they probably weren't aware of the lessons and toughness I'd learned growing up on the court. If they had known, they never would have bet against me.

After years of preparing, I was finally ready to move on to my chosen specialty of urology. I looked forward to taking this final step. With all the challenges and uncertainties I had endured over the years, I wasn't worried about not succeeding. I had been through way too much to fail by this time.

Chapter Sixteen:

THE MICHAEL JORDAN OF UROLOGY

I approached my promotion to urology training mildly nervous, but mostly excited. I had been taught operative technique in general surgery, but I now needed to shape and hone my surgical skills to fit my specialty. My personal goal was to witness and participate in as much as possible. In only three years, I would no longer be in training but the person in charge in the OR, ultimately responsible for anything that happened. I wanted to care for patients with every disease process and be exposed to all possible variations to best prepare for the future. I also wanted to manage (and hopefully not cause) a wide variety of surgical complications while I still had the security of an attending to back me up.

At SUNY Buffalo, the urology attendings were supportive and took their roles as instructors seriously. Our chairman was a rare individual, a true genius, which could be intimidating as he continuously pressed us to grasp complex concepts and recall the literature to support our theories. If a patient had a problem that seemed straightforward, we were required to consider all possibilities rather than assume that the obvious approach was the best. Our chairman was demanding, but we knew he was looking out for our best interests. Similar to my exposure to great coaches and instructors on the court, he not only taught skills that would last—he supplied us with values that would stay with us forever.

Four years of college, four more of medical school, an additional two in general surgery training, and a final three to achieve board certification in urology. It was a long road, yet training in urology was regimented. For example, it was well known which surgical procedure you would be allowed to perform as a first-year urology resident and which would be permitted for each of the following years. However, even if a specific case was appropriate for your level of training, it was still the attending physician's decision to determine whether you were ready and how much you could do independently. Being the primary surgeon was a privilege you needed to earn by demonstrating your dedication and commitment. This wasn't written down anywhere but was passed along from those ahead and picked up from our daily interactions with the staff. Similar to the court, your game minutes were earned by your effort and performance at practice.

Each of the first-year residents in urology had trained at different general surgery programs for the two previous years. I was the only resident my year who had also completed general surgery training at SUNY Buffalo, and my experience prepared me well. The initial year of urology training was as enjoyable as I had anticipated, and more important, for the first time since the early days of medical school, we were treated with respect and even able to have a modest social life. Although we remained on call every night, we were able to cover the patients from home. Still, we were called often and had to return to the hospital frequently. But being able to sleep in your own bed, even if only for part of the night, made all the difference in the world.

At the end of my first year of urology training, I was called to the emergency room to assess a gentleman who was unable to void. His urinary stream had slowed down so much in the past few weeks that he couldn't pass urine at all and presented to the ER in terrible pain.

Mr. Williams was sixty-three years old and had no health insurance or primary care physician. He was incredibly grateful when I arrived at the emergency room and drained over a liter of fluid from his bladder. His kidneys hadn't been able to empty because his prostate was blocking his bladder outlet. As a result, he had developed renal failure and life-threatening electrolyte abnormalities. I spent hours getting him admitted to a cardiac-monitored floor with a lower patient-to-nurse ratio. Correcting his metabolic imbalances was time consuming and required continual fluid resuscitation and adjustment, so it was essential that I be in constant contact with the nursing staff there. After a solid twenty-four to forty-eight hours of this intense activity, his kidneys improved and eventually regained their complete function. His cardiovascular system also required intervention with a variety of medications to maintain optimal performance with the wide fluid shifts that occurred during his resuscitation. Consulting another service to assist with these complex medical issues would have been acceptable for many specialties, but my general surgical training had taught me differently. I felt comfortable managing all his non-urologic problems on my own.

Within several days, Mr. Williams improved greatly and was medically stable. The attending of record determined that he'd require a standard prostate operation known as a TURP (transurethral resection of the prostate) to channel an opening through his prostate and allow him to void normally again. I discussed the procedure with him at length, and he was anxious to have it performed during this hospital stay so he wouldn't have to go home with a tube.

* * *

As a first-year urology resident, I had yet to perform a TURP since this procedure was considered a second-year case. I did, however, have a thorough understanding of the anatomy. I had also read extensively about this procedure, its risks, and its complications, and I had observed many TURPs performed by attending physicians and fellow residents. I had cared for this patient almost exclusively since his admission, and as far as he was concerned, I was his doctor. More specifically, I was his urologist. He was already comfortable with me, and I had earned his trust and confidence. I was ready to be instructed on my first TURP, and he was the ideal candidate. "Put me in, Coach," I thought. "I'm ready to go. I won't disappoint you."

The attending physician on service was considered one of the strongest academics in the program and was also the residency program director. I had gotten along well with him, and since he was younger than most of the other instructors and fairly close to me in age, I considered him both a friend and an adviser. On the day of the scheduled surgery, I personally wheeled Mr. Williams to the operating room and watched as he was transferred to the OR table and placed under general anesthesia. I looked expectantly toward my attending in hopes that I would get the nod to proceed. I was certain he knew exactly what I was thinking since I'd made it obvious in the days leading up to the operation that I was ready.

But the signal never came. As the attending placed the scope into the bladder, my heart sank. It was obvious that once again, I was going to be a bystander. Yet I knew it was my time to prove myself.

Sinking into the realization that my involvement in this case would be minimal, I decided to give it one last shot and straight out asked if I was to be anything more than an observer. The attending gently informed me that I would not because I wasn't officially a second-year urology resident. "Just a few more weeks to go, Bruce. Don't worry, you'll get there soon enough."

His answer didn't make sense based on my skill level and my history with the patient, though, and the unfairness of the situation sent an agonizing fire through my body. I felt comfortable enough with this attending to argue my position, which I did, this time with my voice raised. Again I was denied. Resigned to the inevitable and with overwhelming emotion, I looked my attending in the eye and declared with complete sincerity, "I know it's your decision, but you realize you're keeping Michael Jordan on the bench!"

I didn't know where that line had come from since I had never said it before or even heard it. Deeply disappointed, I stormed off to the recovery room to write the postoperative orders for the patient and to figure out what I would do next. I didn't need to watch this case; I needed to do this case.

While writing the orders, one of the OR nurses ran over to the area where I was sitting and stared at me as she caught her breath. Although she was one of those nurses who had been at the hospital forever, she shook her head and laughed, saying, "Now I've seen it all." She told me I had been asked to come back into the operating room to do the procedure. Apparently, the attending had gotten quite a charge out of my unexpected outburst and had instructed the nurse to grab me and ask that I scrub back into the case. As I walked back into the OR, my attending looked up at me with a huge smile and said, "OK, Michael, let's see what you can do."

As you can imagine, I was all too eager to accept the challenge and demonstrate my skills. The case ended up being exciting and fun with a successful patient outcome.

Years later, I saw this same attending give a lecture in Worcester, Massachusetts, where I was in practice at the time. Unexpectedly, he announced to the audience, "We are all honored to have the Michael Jordan of urology in the crowd this evening."

As often was the case on the court, sometimes you just need an opportunity to make things happen.

SUNY Buffalo had three urology residents per year for the three-year program. Therefore, at any one time, there were nine residents in training. You would start as a junior resident, then become a senior resident the next year and finally a chief resident. Since we had eight hospitals to cover on any given day, there usually weren't enough residents to assist on the major cases. This resulted in an outstanding operative experience and was probably what attracted me most to the program. We also had fellows being trained in the program. These physicians had finished their chief year in urology and were now performing an extra year of training to further their expertise.

As a junior and senior resident, you would spend three-month rotations at the VA Hospital, where you were given a lot of responsibility and expected to work fairly independently. The fellow on rotation, usually having trained at a different program, would be in charge of running the service. The residents all looked forward to this rotation as the patients were appreciative, the pathology was diverse, and the attendings were helpful without being overly demanding.

Early in the rotation, a fifty-eight-year-old man presented to the urology clinic after experiencing several episodes of thick blood in his urine. The fellow assessed him and ordered the appropriate studies, which revealed a medium-sized mass in the left kidney, more than likely a cancerous growth. He recommended removing the kidney, and the procedure was scheduled. As it was the start of the fellow's new position, he was excited to perform this complex operation and had handpicked the attending surgeon, knowing he would let him perform most of the case.

This attending, a community urologist with academic ties, was well liked among the residents and fellows because he was competent, down-to-earth, and respectful. The nursing staff also loved working with him but for different reasons. He was always on time and extremely fast in the operating room—two qualities they cherished above all others. Since this would be the fellow's first nephrectomy at this program, he had tended to all the details personally and couldn't wait to proceed. He was ready to prove himself and establish a solid reputation.

As a senior resident, I was to be the second assist, which meant that I did little other than hold retractors so everyone else could see. The junior resident, a good friend of mine, would be observing way down at the end of the table where he would barely be able to see anything, but he was still expected to be there. I figured that in addition to holding retractors, my other task was to keep the junior resident from falling asleep by joking under my breath or rolling my eyes when the fellow and the attending were trying to act cool. When it came down to it, I wasn't doing much more than he was.

The case went smoothly, completed in record time even for this particular attending. The fellow was pleased, taking most of the credit for having just removed his first kidney at a new hospital, skillfully and with minimal blood loss. The attending left us to close the incision, politely thanked all in the room, and said to call him if he was needed for anything, since he probably would not come back to this hospital for months. Then he was out the door long before the patient was to be transferred to the recovery room.

As residents, we were expected to write the post-op orders, take care of the patient while he was hospitalized, and follow up at the clinic after discharge. We were pleased to be finished so quickly as we had a ton of work with our inpatients on the floor. Maybe we would even get home at a reasonable hour. As we began wrapping up the case, we were all laughing and joking and congratulating the fellow, who was proud he'd made a tough case look easy. He told us he was ready for his next challenge and hoped he'd soon be allowed to take the residents through cases by himself. However, for that honor, we knew he'd have to earn the confidence of the attending staff. Today was a good first step.

Beep, beep, beep, beep, b-e-e-e-e-e-p .....

The tone of the room drastically changed as the monitors shrilled with horror. The anesthesiologist looked up, flushed and panic-stricken. As the patient was being transferred from the OR table to the stretcher, his blood pressure had plummeted to dangerously low levels. Since the surgery had gone so smoothly, our first thought was that something must be wrong with the monitors. But the man's repeated manual vital signs confirmed the extreme hypotension. This guy was fading fast, and we didn't know why.

At the fellow's direction, the nurses frantically tried calling the attending, but he was long gone. With the patient's blood pressure critical and no other surgeon present, the fellow recited the differential diagnosis and considered what to do next. We kept the patient on the table and rapidly reviewed the options, as the fellow stat paged the attending without success. It was now up to him to determine the next course of action.

With several monitors screeching in unison, the fellow exclaimed that the patient was experiencing a massive myocardial infarction and needed to be taken to the ICU and treated by medicine. He then yelled at the junior resident and me to move our patient onto the stretcher and get him out of the OR as quickly as possible. I looked at my buddy. Without speaking, we acknowledged that the fellow's conclusion was probably not correct. So I told him that we suspected a massive bleed and recommended exploring the abdomen immediately. The fellow yelled back that we were wrong and that because he was the ranking physician in the room as well as the surgeon of record, the patient should be transferred out. When I challenged him again on his decision, he impatiently reiterated his directives and left the OR.

Exasperated, we prepared to move the patient, but his blood pressure was no longer registering, despite anesthesia administering large amounts of fluids and medication to keep the pressure up. If this situation persisted any longer, the patient was going to die.

With the situation now critical and the fellow absent, I decided I was the ranking surgeon and took charge. After a brief exchange with my junior, whose surgical instincts I trusted, we agreed to open the incision against the direct orders of our superior. We felt so certain about our decision that we were ready to take the heat if we were wrong.

"Make a decision. It may not be right, but make one and stand by it," rose up from my years of general surgery training. We were ready to go this alone.

We splashed iodine onto the abdomen and with a hemostat, we hastily removed the skin staples, which flew in all directions. Without hesitating, we incised the strongly sutured fascia with heavy scissors in one quick motion. The wound sprung open, and liters of blood overflowed from the peritoneal cavity, overwhelming the suction equipment. This made it difficult to isolate the cause of the massive bleed, so we threw numerous lap pads into the wound to absorb the flow.

Assuming this rapid and heavy bleeding could only be coming from the main renal artery where the kidney had been removed, I explored the area, feeling the pulsating aorta and running my fingers along the vessel until I found the source of the bleeding.

My assumption had been right. I applied pressure to the spot and watched I frantically suctioned out the remaining pooled blood. The surgical ties had blown off, and there was now a free flow of blood directly from the aorta into the wound. After we isolated the bleeding area and suture-ligated the pumping vessel, the junior resident and I irrigated the abdomen and closed the wound again. The patient would require several units of blood, but we knew that he was stable now.

Opening the patient and exploring his abdomen had proved to be the correct decision. If we'd waited even a few more minutes, he probably would have died.

As we were closing the abdomen for the second time, the fellow came back into the operating room to find out why we hadn't made it to recovery. We filled him in on what happened which was relayed to the attending later that day.

I believe there are defining moments in our lives and our careers. For my residency, that event was mine. Word of the incident spread quickly throughout the program, and that evening during a social gathering, our peers treated the junior resident and me like celebrities. The other residents wanted to know the details, which we shared many times throughout the night. We were careful, however, not to let the attending urologists know who did exactly what. They had heard some rumblings about an "exciting case" that day but didn't know the details. We didn't want to further damage the fellow's reputation; unfortunately, his defining moment would take him a while to overcome. He eventually did, but it was difficult and demonstrated how initial impressions are almost impossible to change.

It was still early in my year as a senior resident, but I was counting the days until I'd become a chief. I knew I was ready.

Chapter Seventeen:

WHEN IN DOUBT, STICK IT WITH A NEEDLE

In my chief year of training, I could finally see the light at the end of the very long tunnel. I was so accustomed to the routine now that although work was extensive, it was manageable, despite being on call every night. Privileges came with the responsibilities of being chief, most notably choosing which operative cases you would be involved with the next day and assigning the other cases to those more junior. Some you were obligated to cover, but you could often choose to assist a urologist at a smaller hospital with the more interesting or complex cases. The residents looked forward to these opportunities, since for the most part the attendings were very supportive and appreciated our assistance. If you demonstrated confidence in your abilities or if the attending lacked confidence in his own, you'd be allowed to perform most of the operation, which was a great experience. The situation at these outlying hospitals gave residents the chance to be exposed to many approaches to the same surgical procedures in a fairly low-stress environment.

My schedule was open when I was called to assist an attending physician with a right nephrectomy. We would be performing the procedure on a seventy-two-year-old man to remove a renal mass suspected of being cancer. I had not met this attending before, but I had heard good things about him from my colleagues, and I agreed to help out. I'd also been told this doctor used an anterior chevron approach, which uses an incision through the abdomen rather than the flank. I found this less common approach unnecessarily tedious, but I wanted to see the anatomy it would reveal and thought it would be a good experience. The case was scheduled to start at

7:30 a.m., but I arrived thirty minutes late due to an emergency with one of my own patients at another hospital that demanded my full attention and took precedence. I had called into the operating room to let the attending know what was going on, but apparently that wasn't good enough. As this was my first visit to this hospital, I also had trouble finding parking, locating the locker room, and getting a pair of scrubs.

When I finally arrived and stepped into the OR, the attending surgeon had already started the case with assistance from his senior associate. I introduced myself, apologized for my tardiness, and again explained the emergency that had kept me from being on time. They both grunted in response. "You can scrub in . . . if you want," the attending said.

I got the impression these guys believed they were doing me a great favor by allowing me to observe them and thought I should be more appreciative of their invitation. I considered leaving but decided to scrub in anyway to avoid burning any bridges for my future. Maybe they'd teach me something, too; I had nothing else planned anyway.

After I was completely scrubbed and gowned, the circulating nurse told me that I had contaminated myself by touching something unsterile and that I needed to repeat my scrub. Wow, what level of training did she think I was at? Asking me to rescrub was the kind of nonsense pulled on a first-year medical student, certainly not a chief resident in line to graduate within the next few months. It was an old-school tactic I saw early on in my training. Under the guise of protecting sterility, scrub nurses would often make a student or young resident scrub a second or even third time, claiming there had been a breach in protocol. A scrub nurse and family friend who had been at MCV for over twenty-five years told me this had nothing to do with sterility but was meant to embarrass and assert authority. In this case, I was well aware that the nurse was just following the lead of the attendings. I found her audacity amusing and laughed to myself as I walked back into the OR after scrubbing a second time. This should be interesting, I thought.

When I returned, I was given the second assist's position, meaning my only responsibility was holding

retractors. The two associates were obviously per-
turbed that I had the gall to show up late and didn't
even acknowledge my presence for another forty-five
minutes, all the while laughing it up with the staff. I
strained to watch the two of them work, mostly to be
polite and look interested, as they isolated and tied off
the renal artery.

I was finally addressed when I tried more aggres-
sively to peer into the wound, at which point I was
just trying not to fall asleep on my feet. "Just to get
you up to speed, Bruce, here's the kidney, and we can
palpate this large mass. Here's the renal artery, which
we have already tied off nicely, and this is the renal
vein, which we are about to divide. Classic case, and it
has only now been an hour and fifteen minutes since
we started. Too bad you showed up late."

I was then allowed to move to the front and
look into the wound to see exactly what they were
describing. Immediately a pang of horror hit me as I
realized what they were about to do. "That's not the
renal vein. That's the duodenum," I calmly stated,
despite how I felt inside. This was the first time I'd
spoken since scrubbing back in, and it didn't make

the two seasoned surgeons very happy. The duodenum is the first portion of the small intestine, and if resected like they had told me they were about to do, the patient would become very sick and possibly die.

These surgeons, who had been in practice for over fifty years combined, were still seething over my late appearance. Their egos wouldn't allow them to believe they could make such an obvious error. The younger attending, clearly angered by my perceived insolence, proceeded to put a large clamp on this structure that I had warned them about. At this point, I didn't care what they thought of me; I had made up my mind to try to help the poor patient out since he had no control of his own fate. "I know that's the duodenum," I said. "I'm sure that the vein is in there somewhere, and if you like, I can help you find it."

The two grew even more annoyed and gave me a patronizing, nonsensical explanation of why I was wrong.

"OK," I said, "I dare you to put a needle into it. Either way, it won't do any harm, but we'll know what we're dealing with. If it's the renal vein, blood should return, and if not, then there'll be something green and you'll also know what's going on. If I'm wrong, I promise to keep my mouth shut."

The surgeons reluctantly agreed and asked the staff to bring in a 10cc syringe they could attach to a small needle. When one of the surgeons finally inserted the needle and pulled back, a thick, greenish substance accompanied by gas returned as I had expected, indicating the small intestine and not the renal vein. The surgeon then frantically removed the clamp, identified and tied off the true renal vein, and completed the operation.

When a surgical procedure is performed with the assistance of a resident, the resident is expected to accompany the patient to the recovery room, write the postoperative orders, and be certain that the patient is stable before leaving the area. This usually takes an extra thirty minutes and frees up the attending to do other work or, more commonly, hang out with buddies and go to lunch. However, in this case, I was told before the abdomen was closed that I would be excused since I "must be so busy with the university guys." I never saw those doctors again, and they never called me back to assist them. Even if they had, I would have declined.

That incident was another defining moment in my career. At that point, I knew I was ready to be out on my own and begin practice as a full attending. I had a lot more to learn and knew medical education was an ongoing process, but I was ready to be the one in charge. Our chairman had accomplished his goal: he had trained another capable urologist. I was eager to graduate, join real-world medicine, and help some people.

But there was a problem. A major change was occurring in our country, one that involved oil and war and could affect me greatly. At age thirty-two, I might find myself in the military.

Chapter Eighteen:

READY TO SERVE

As I walked into the room to attend our weekly urology conference at the VA Hospital, I was greeted by two very serious men in full military attire and a whole lot of decorations on their chests.

"You must be Dr. Rosenfeld?" They asked to speak with the three chief residents and knew each of us by name. The country had just moved into Iraq for the first Gulf War, and no one knew how much the conflict would escalate. I was about to complete my residency in general and trauma surgery with a specialization in urology. I was ready to become independent after working so hard for the past five years, but the United States government had something else in mind.

The recruiters informed each of the chief residents of the possibility of being drafted into the army. They said that if the conflict turned into a full-blown war, the armed forces would have enough physicians to cover only 40 percent of their needs. They then went on to describe the inevitable special doctor's draft and explained to us that all physicians were eligible until age forty-five.

"The first doctors taken are those who have most recently finished their residency and have a surgical background, especially if they're experienced in trauma surgery." In other words, the three of us were about as high up in the draft as possible, and we should expect to be summoned if the war intensified. I wasn't afraid, but I did want to be pragmatic and act logically.

At this time, I had been married for four years to Lisa, whom I met when I was a fourth-year student at the Medical College of Virginia, where she had just begun her training in pediatrics. Despite her being incredibly busy during her internship, we were able to spend enough time together to figure out that this was the real thing. Lisa was able to transfer from MCV and complete her residency at SUNY Buffalo so that we could be together, an incredible sacrifice on her part. We made it through these busy years with our marriage intact, although at the beginning, with my being on call every other night and her every third, we basically watched each other sleep when we were home at the same time. This schedule wasn't easy on a young marriage, but we managed to get through it fairly unscathed and were ready to start a real life together without the massive time constraints.

With this unexpected potential military obligation, Lisa and I didn't know whether we should look for jobs in other cities, buy a house, or make any plans at all. We did know that if I was called to duty, we couldn't afford a mortgage, as we already had substantial medical school loans to repay. We weren't afraid of what the future held, but we did need some information so that we could make reasonable plans.

Not all the chiefs reacted the same way I did. When the army officers first approached us, one of my fellow chief residents was overwhelmed and nearly broke down. My friend had extensive family and financial obligations awaiting him in his hometown, and being called into military service didn't fit into his plans at all. We leaned on each other quite a bit for the following few weeks, and over time, he adjusted to the possibilities. After the initial shock wore off, all of us decided we would do whatever was required to assist the military since we had the necessary training. We would serve without complaint, taking this unexpected commitment one day at a time. After all, there was no use getting upset about something over which we had zero control.

As it turned out, the first Gulf War was short, and the military never required our service. It was an interesting time in our training, however, and it was even more fascinating to look back on our reactions. We were ready to serve; the final call just never came.

Chapter Nineteen:

HOOP DREAMS

I woke up in a cold sweat, completely drained. My heart was pounding so hard that I wondered if I was actually having a heart attack. Frightened but strangely exhilarated, I slowly realized I was in my own bed and had just experienced a recurring dream, one that often leaves me soaking wet and in pain from the physical activity.

There's always some minor variation; this time the coach was calling for me to get into the game, but I couldn't find my basketball shoes. I went crazy looking for something to put on my feet but couldn't find anything. Not wanting to miss the opportunity to play, I ran to cover my assigned player, who quickly sped his way up the court. I tried my best to catch up to him, but with only socks on my feet, I couldn't gain traction and ended up falling to my knees, frustrated and humiliated. This time it was a horrible experience, but other times, I make the winning shot and am swept up by a wave of teammates and fans in a moment of sheer joy.

I've had these dreams about once a month since age eleven. I have never been trained in interpretation, but knowing how deeply basketball is ingrained in my being and the influence it still has over me, the dream doesn't seem too hard to figure out. Even today when I'm just shooting around on a basketball court, I listen to the sounds from within my body and can feel the rhythm of the game. I'm always comforted by the familiarity of it all.

Having completed my training, I now had much more free time. I was still relatively young and figured it might be a good point to get back into basketball. Even though I'd played in only a handful of pickup games during my residency, I didn't think it would be too difficult to get into shape again and recover my skills to a respectable level. I was excited when I was asked to play ball with a bunch of guys who'd been meeting every Sunday for years.

Their ages ranged widely, but I was one of the youngest. In the past, if a player was even approaching thirty, we thought he was crazy for wanting to play, and we tried not to hurt him. Despite this long-held belief of mine, I was ready to get on the court again and have some fun.

As I walked into the gym located in a small church, I could hear the rhythm of the bouncing ball and the squeal of basketball shoes on the freshly waxed floor. I was elated. I noticed that the players interacted well and seemed like a good bunch of guys, and I couldn't wait to regain at least a small part of what I had once loved.

After a short wait, it was my team's turn to play. The ball was passed inbounds to me, and I quickly established myself as the point guard of this five-man unit. I dribbled the ball across the half-court line and instinctively looked at the defense to assess my options. The guy covering me was several years older and a bit taller, with the confidence of someone who had played at a fairly high level at one point in his life. As I pushed the ball up the court, I looked directly at him and could tell from the way he shuffled his feet that he didn't have my speed (or the speed I thought I still had). From there, my decision was second nature, as it had been so many times in the past. Drive left, flip the ball behind my back right to shake off my man, and split the defender playing down low and covering my buddy. Option 1: if the defense comes up on me, dish it off for an assist. Option 2: if the defense stays put, continue up the middle for a soft layin. I had done it thousands of times before, and I could make an impact with this first play to establish a presence for the rest of this game and for any in the future. I was ready, confident that the result would be a basket.

Driving to the left was easy, but after that, things didn't go so smoothly. I lost the ball on the simple behind-the-back, and it bounced out of bounds. I then tried other, less complex moves, and none of them seemed to work either. I had no timing and couldn't make a basket to save my life. My mind could envision what I was supposed to do, but my body didn't respond. This wasn't fun anymore.

In the past, I never had to think about playing the game. Every move was a definitive action when attacking or an innate reaction to a given situation. I had great confidence in my body and my skills, and if the game came down to the last play, I wanted the ball in my hands so I could be the person who took the final shot. In most cases, my teammates were fine with this as well.

As I sat on the sideline awaiting a chance for us to redeem ourselves after losing our first game, I watched the teams now playing and thought they looked like a bunch of old men out there. It didn't take me long to realize that my skills were no better. As a direct result of my experience that day, I decided it was time to give it up. Basketball had lost its appeal, and playing at this level was just too frustrating. Good decision? Bad decision? I wasn't sure. That's just the way it was.

After describing the experience to one of my physician buddies who'd known me when I was much younger and still able to play, he taunted me repeatedly. "Rosenfeld, you're a has-been. You're left with nothing." He was right in some ways, but at the same time, he was very wrong. Basketball had been a huge part of my development, and he was correct in that I no longer had the skills to play at the level I wanted to. But I knew that the game was firmly within me, and the lessons I'd learned could be summoned in any situation.

One of the greatest gifts basketball gave me is the ability to pick myself up after a failure or a suboptimal performance and move on. More succinctly, it taught me how to turn a negative into a positive, as a good friend of mine likes to proclaim. The skills I had learned from the game allowed me to get through the peaks and valleys of becoming a physician and a surgeon.

Throughout basketball training, I can't tell you how often we heard the "You don't appreciate the value of this ball" speech, which at one point we could all recite almost verbatim. The motivational talk starts with the coach placing a basketball at the free-throw line and standing behind it. "I can go out today and replace this ball for twenty-five dollars, but if you think that's what this ball is truly worth, you're very wrong." He would then go on to tell us about the chance for a full ride to college and the tens of thousands of dollars that a scholarship was worth, as well as the doors that would open for us afterward. Being typical self-absorbed teenagers, we usually listened to the lecture with eyes glazed over, thinking our coaches had no idea what they were talking about. But these coaches were completely right, even more than they would ever know in my case.

Basketball taught me values and gave me principles that allowed me to be accepted by a competitive college, attend medical school, and become a surgeon. It taught me discipline, patience in learning, mental toughness in the face of adversity, and the ability to bounce back from a failed effort. Not a bad return for a twenty-five-dollar investment.

Early in my career as an attending surgeon, I was involved in a very difficult surgical procedure. The patient had a large bladder tumor that was invading the muscle wall, and the proper treatment was to remove the entire bladder and fashion a new bladder out of the small intestine. Usually, this is a six-to-eight-hour operation, depending on the scarring and the patient's body habitus. This poor guy was only in his late sixties, but he was obese, had an extensive smoking history, and, as we later found out, was an alcoholic.

Initially, the patient did well postoperatively, but he later developed an intestinal leak where I had anastomosed two ends back together after isolating a segment to create a new bladder. The complication required a second operation to resect the area and reattach the bowel. I liked this patient and felt bad, even guilty, that he'd had a rocky course. He had severe disease and poor nutrition and was at high risk for this problem, yet I still took this complication to heart.

Intellectually, I knew that if you performed enough cases, you would encounter complications no matter how great your surgical skills, but I was having a lot of trouble accepting this in my own practice. Despite the many years I'd spent in training, I had not learned my lessons about dealing with disappointment as well as I should have. It was my wife who set me straight, firmly reminding me of a truism I've never forgotten: "If you can't deal with the complications, you can't be a surgeon. We can't go through this every time there's a problem."

She was right, and despite being fortunate enough to have had minimal surgical complications in my practice, remembering these words allows me to better deal with them as they occur. I'd learned from my basketball training how not to get down on myself, but on occasion I needed a boost that Lisa was great at providing.

Although I now had the extra time to do the things I had neglected over the years, basketball no longer was a priority for me. I just couldn't get any enjoyment out of playing the game at a level so far below where I had been just a few years ago. My shot was lousy, I couldn't get up anywhere near the rim, and dribbling no longer felt natural but like a chore. Surprisingly, I wasn't bothered too much saying goodbye to the game and moving on to other athletic endeavors. I took up running and would eventually complete three full marathons. I still had great memories of basketball and was lucky enough to have come away from the game with values that would last me a lifetime. I was fortunate for other reasons, too. I still had my dreams, and in most of those games, I haven't lost a step.

Chapter Twenty:

THE PRIVILEGE OF BEING A DOCTOR

After completing our residencies, my wife and I both joined a large multispecialty group practice in Worcester, Massachusetts, and settled into a comfortable house in a nearby town. Being part of a large group allowed me to stay busy from the day I arrived, which is important for a newly trained surgeon. I was confident in my abilities but never missed an opportunity to learn from my senior associates. I constantly bombarded them with questions regarding specific cases. The group also had the distinction of being affiliated with the University of Massachusetts Medical School, so as I moved into practice on my own, I had the responsibility and privilege of training urology residents.

Being an instructor to residents was a highlight for me, and I quickly realized that one needs a much greater understanding to teach than to perform a procedure. I came to recognize that anyone can perform surgery, but if you can teach someone else, you're at the next level. In this sense, my education continued, and I was proud of that accomplishment.

Shortly after arriving at the group practice, I was asked to see a seventy-two-year-old gentleman for dark clotted blood in his urine. Jim was evaluated with a CT scan, which revealed a kidney mass larger than a football. Amazingly, he was not in any pain, and his only symptoms were minor night sweats and weight loss. A full metastatic workup was negative for any disease outside the area of the kidney, but the mass did extend well into the liver and promised to be extremely challenging to remove.

Rarely had I found the need for assistance, but with a mass of this size, I thought it appropriate to ask for the help of a surgical oncologist, a good friend of mine with whom, coincidentally, I had played ball many years before at MCV when he was a resident. The case went well, and we successfully removed the large cancerous mass.

Incredibly, Jim's hospital stay lasted only five days, and directly after the surgery, he insisted he felt great. I've heard many times that large tumors just make a patient feel lousy all over. This gentleman was seen several times in follow–up, and once he was cleared medically, he said he was ready to embark on a few trips that he had put off.

The pathology demonstrated that this was an aggressive kidney cancer, but various scans gave no evidence that it had spread to the surrounding lymph nodes or other organs, at this time in medicine, there was nothing else to do. Due to the size and aggressive nature of the mass, we weren't overly optimistic about Jim's long-term prognosis, but we did not want to discourage him from participating in any activities he felt ready for. We had no idea how much time he had left and knew that his upcoming vacation was important to him.

Jim's operation was in January, and after the initial postoperative period, I didn't hear back from him until mid-November, when he presented to the emergency room with severe back pain. It had begun as mild discomfort three to four weeks earlier, but in the last few days, it had become unbearable. A thorough evaluation traced the pain to metastatic disease. The cancer had spread to his spine, eating away at the bone and causing the vertebrae to collapse on themselves. A bone scan revealed that most of the spine was now involved, along with many other bones.

While hospitalized, Jim was treated for his pain and put on a regimen of morphine pills. He was then allowed to go home, only to return several weeks later in even more pain and with a number of new issues. His remaining kidney was blocked by the cancer, and there were very few areas of his body not involved. Realizing the futility of any further experimental or heroic treatment, he elected to simply be treated with narcotics to try to keep his pain under control while his organ systems began to permanently shut down.

Late one evening, as I was sitting by Jim's bedside on an unusually quiet hospital floor, I listened to Jim describe his emotions, as he had only days or perhaps even hours to live. Amazingly, he was at great peace. I believe this was thanks to his faith, which gave him the strength to await death with such dignity. I admired his courage and took the opportunity to ask him if the extensive surgical procedure I'd performed only ten months before had been a waste. He was passionate and emotional in his response, explaining that he had spent the last nine months traveling, visiting relatives he'd not seen in years and essentially saying goodbye. He was appreciative for that opportunity and said that until the last few weeks, he'd actually felt pretty good.

When he eventually passed on, I cried to myself and felt an emptiness inside. It wouldn't be the last time I would have that feeling. I have always thought that with each patient's death, a little of me dies as well. I know it sounds cliché, but it truly feels this way. I believe that experiencing that sense of loss helps keep me human. I don't want to lose that feeling. It makes me work harder to help those I can.

This is part of the true privilege of being a physician, and I hope never to take it for granted. It means seeing people at the end of their lives and trying to help them through the most difficult of challenges. I admire the peace and dignity with which some people proceed through the end of their lives. I marvel at their inner strength and don't know if I would react the same in similar circumstances.

On more than one occasion, I have told a patient how shortchanged I felt in not having known them when they weren't ill, seeing how strong and in control they were in the worst of situations. I could only imagine what they were like when things were good. I have seen the power of family and the power of faith many times over, and the stories are inspiring.

Thomas was a sixty-two-year-old man who never liked going to doctors. He thought he was a little overweight but otherwise healthy, and he came to me because of recent difficultly voiding associated with some minor low-back pain. As part of my evaluation, I ordered a PSA level. A PSA is a blood test that helps screen for prostate cancer by measuring the amount of prostate-specific antigen, a protein produced in the prostate gland. A normal level is less than 4.0 in most situations, but his was well over 500. A needle biopsy of his prostate confirmed he had an aggressive form of prostate cancer, and metastatic workup showed that this cancer had already spread throughout his body.

He was treated with hormonal therapy, which dropped his PSA to less than 1.0, indicating a quick remission. We were all very happy. He was voiding better, and his back pain had disappeared. For several months, Thomas did well—that is, until the pain predictably returned to his spine and required hospitalization. Scans showed that the remission had been short lived; the cancer was now even more extensive. While lying in his hospital bed, he had a seizure, and a brain MRI demonstrated numerous tumors consistent with the prostate cancer migrating to the area. Thomas's medical team then consulted a neurologist to help get his seizures under control.

In a few months, this man went from being a robust, hardworking, slightly overweight but otherwise healthy person to not being able to lift his head from his pillow. He knew he was going to die soon, but he pleaded with me to try my best to keep him alive for just a few more days.

"My daughter is studying in London, and she's flying home on Sunday. Bruce, you're my man, the guy I rely on. Just keep me alive long enough to say goodbye to her. I need to do that. She's my only daughter."

I left that conversation with tears in my eyes, which I hid from the nursing staff and the family, and worked around the clock to keep him going until his daughter arrived. Thomas did get to see his daughter for several hours until he was too weak to interact. Later that evening he passed away. I never underestimate the power of love and family.

After numerous encounters like this over the years, I began to concentrate on treating prostate disease and prostate cancer. I believed this area of urology deserved great consideration and compassion from the urologist, and I thought I could do it right. I tried to approach every patient with respect and dignity, always being realistic but never extinguishing hope. I learned that I should never push any particular procedure or therapy onto a patient and that the treatment decision must be made together. Over the years I also learned the importance of quality of life and that one can live a lifetime in three months or six months or any amount of time, taking each day as if it were your last.

When I was caring for patients in the ICU during my training, I came to learn that some conditions are much worse than death. I'm thinking specifically of cases where patients creep in and out of consciousness while on complete life support and have intermittent bouts of sepsis, only to eventually succumb to multisystem organ failure. During my training we kept countless people alive until the family requested us to stop. I know that the decision to remove support was heart-wrenching for the family; I can only hope the patients didn't suffer too much in the meantime.

These examples are just two of the hundreds and maybe thousands of similar experiences I have had during my years of practice. This is why we as physicians get up each morning and go to work despite having to deal with the ever-increasing nonsense of government regulation and insurance company aggravation that has been forced on our profession. We have been entrusted to be in the unique position to make a difference in the lives of those around us. Whether it is saving a life or easing pain, I never forget that we have the ability and the potential to make a difference. To me, this is the true privilege of being a physician, and those in our profession, and society as a whole, should never downplay its importance or take it for granted. It allows you to meet incredibly strong and inspirational people all the time, like Jay, who has turned out to be one of my favorite patients.

Jay was a healthy fifty-year-old who had been a basketball star while at a small college in the Midwest. He moved to Tucson at age twenty-eight to work in a law firm and was a highly regarded professional who kept himself trim and in excellent condition. His genuine enthusiasm for life, positive nature, and athletic physique belied his age. He was driven and used to facing problems head-on, and he believed in the strength of the individual. Jay worked out regularly and went to his primary care physician for an annual routine examination. With his fifty-year milestone, it was time to start preventive screening for a number of diseases, so his doctor ordered PSA screening for prostate cancer.

Jay's first PSA test came back at over 9.0, which is considered very high for his age and markedly increased the likelihood of having prostate cancer. So I performed a biopsy, whose results showed a fairly aggressive form of prostate cancer. I was worried about whether it had spread, but we were encouraged when the CT and bone scans showed no sign of metastatic disease. Now it was time to talk to Jay again. This conversation was particularly difficult for me, probably because he was so easy for me to relate to. He was a young, former college athlete who had done everything right and yet now had a bad disease. Despite his misfortune, he remained upbeat and strong and was ready to take on whatever he had to fight it.

Two or three times a week, I would sit down with a patient, usually accompanied by his spouse, to tell him we found prostate cancer on a biopsy. When I was younger, it wasn't that hard a task. I went through describing the disease process, answered all questions, and made my recommendations. I was always patient and respectful, but delivering the news didn't bother me in a personal way like it does now.

As I've gotten older, this conversation has become harder for me. It usually lasts more than an hour; we draw pictures and talk about the risks and benefits of all possible options, and then I recommend that the patient visit websites and read books to become better educated. Over the years, I've gotten very good at this conversation. I never take any of these encounters lightly but have found a way to present all of the options in a succinct, understandable, and organized manner so that the patients come out well informed and with a good idea of what their next steps should be. Rarely does anyone leave my office feeling down, since I always try to instill in them hope and positive thinking, which I think play an important role in the patient's outcome. I want the patient to leave my office thinking, "I've got this disease, but I also have the tools to figure out how best to conquer it and someone who'll be by my side the whole way." Most important to me is that I never want him to feel he's alone in this fight.

"We'll get through this together" is one of the sincere statements I make during this conversation, reaching back to the well-learned team concept from my training years. I see my role as the ultimate patient advocate and educator. Despite my being a surgeon, it's obvious that surgery isn't the only treatment for this type of cancer, and we review all the options. I honestly tell patients that in my career I have performed so many surgical procedures to remove the prostate that I couldn't care less if I perform another. If they choose that option, I'm happy to assist them, but I emphasize that I'm not a young surgeon trying to make a name for myself. I know my skills and also my limitations, and my overall goal is to make sure my patients are happy with their own decisions about treatment. I think my patients like that part of my counsel, and I hope they understand that their absolute best care and cure is my only objective.

Most important in informing a patient that he has prostate cancer is to always speak at a level he can understand and is comfortable with. Over the years, you learn to read a patient's face to see if what you are saying is getting through to him and adjust your approach as needed. I have many patients who are physicians, and the discussions I have with them are much different from those with patients who may be less educated or even intellectually impaired. It has never been difficult for me to tailor this talk to my audience, possibly because I grew up in the public school system, where I was exposed to kids from many backgrounds and of varying cognitive abilities.

I walked into the room and sat in a chair next to Jay to go over his treatment options. We reviewed all his studies, and I told him that his cancer was extensive but that we had found no evidence that it had spread outside the prostate. His choices were radiation and surgery, with a number of subgroups of each. I went over all of these possibilities and discussed the risks and side effects of each, encouraging him, as I do with all my patients, to ask questions.

Jay didn't want to read any books about prostate cancer or look up any information on the websites I'd told him about. He patiently listened to my entire talk and at the end said, "Doc, you were a point guard, right? So you had to tell all your teammates what they had to do and where they had to be. Well, now you're my point guard. You're going to tell me how we're going to beat this, and I know we will. You'll get me through this. I'm not worried."

Ten years later, Jay's still in good shape and working out regularly, without evidence of any disease. This is what makes me happiest in my profession. This, without a doubt, is the true privilege of being a physician.

Chapter Twenty-One:

THE SOUL OF A PHYSICIAN

As a physician, I don't believe that my story is unique. I may be one of the few doctors who discovered he was destined to practice medicine by perfecting ballhandling skills, but most people who were successful in medical school had to learn about dedication and focus at some point in their lives.

Coach Knight is credited with having said, "Most people have the will to win; few have the will to prepare to win." The essential nature of preparation is what Coach Knight taught all of us, even as far back as the summer of 1971, when I was a thirteen-year-old camper at West Point Academy.

Due to the arduous training programs set up by those who orchestrated the American medical education system almost one hundred years ago, most people on their way to becoming doctors have had to overcome a great deal of adversity, if for no other reason than the time commitment of the process. I believe the rigorous course was designed not only to select those who can intellectually handle the program but also to be certain that those who eventually complete the training are emotionally strong enough to deal with the overbearing pressures inherent to the profession.

From the first day of cadaver lab, medical students deal with life-and-death issues that can challenge them to their core. Initially, these assignments are abstract, but in a few years, a name and a face and a family are attached to the disease process, along with the misery and death it may have caused. There were no classes or instruction on how to deal with the emotional reactions of patients or their families.

And certainly there was never any instruction or support in dealing with your own response. Since doctors are part of a highly select group considered academically gifted, we are expected to be strong enough to work through these difficult emotional issues on our own. Ultimately some can't, and this inability to cope may be responsible for the higher rate of substance abuse among physicians than laypeople. As we completed our training, none of us ever had the time or inclination to assess whether this assumption about handling our own emotions was fair or reasonable, but these were the expectations placed on us.

Medicine in general was difficult enough, but in a way, surgery was more challenging because surgeons, like pilots, soldiers, and police officers, are trained to have an exaggerated sense of toughness and aggressiveness so they can make any necessary split-second decisions. If you couldn't handle the stress in training, that was fine from our attending's perspective, since it helped weed out those who didn't have what it takes to become a fully trained surgeon. Anyone can take out an appendix, but can you do this after being awake for forty-eight hours straight? How many patients can you resuscitate in one night before it starts to impair your confidence and effectiveness?

On the basketball court, I learned the importance of study, dedication, repetition, devotion, teaching, being a role model, and believing in my own abilities—lessons that carried me on to become a physician and a surgeon. Because I grew up at the playground and on the basketball court, I was fortunate to have incorporated the skills to be successful to study medicine and even more fortunate to have learned who I was and what I had the potential to do. This relation became apparent to me only when my daughter and I started working on her game as she tried out for her high school freshman team.

It was September of her freshman year, and I felt touched by an angel when out of nowhere my daughter asked, "Hey, Dad, I think I want to go out for the basketball team. Will you teach me how to play?" I was speechless. I had never pushed basketball on her at any time, but I was very excited to start.

We began with the basics: elbows in, fingertips on the ball, and always follow through. My daughter persisted, and as a close relative pointed out, "It looks like the genes have finally kicked in, Bruce." I cherished every moment on the court with my daughter. As we practiced drills and spent hours shooting together, memories lying dormant for decades came streaming back, and I related the stories to my daughter. She was entertained and amused, but she also encouraged me to record my memories in a journal. Taking her advice, I put these accounts on paper and quickly came to understand that the experiences were of greater significance to my development than I had realized. Basketball had been much more than a game, and as a result, my time on the court with my daughter became the inspiration for this book.

My road to becoming a physician and a surgeon was difficult, pushing me to incredibly high levels academically, intellectually, emotionally, and often physically. It required extreme mental and physical discipline to reach this position and fulfill the demands of the profession today. I truly believe that it's an honor and a privilege to be a physician, and I am thankful for all the opportunities and relationships that it has afforded me. I also believe that in large part, my basketball experience taught me the traits and skills necessary to those achievements. I look back with a deep appreciation on all those who helped me attain my goal, in particular the coaches and role models who helped shape my character. I am thankful that basketball taught me to stare a challenge in the eye without blinking and to pursue my dreams no matter who thought it was appropriate to discourage me. Through basketball training, I was taught to trust my instincts, work hard, and try to always do the right thing, knowing there will be times when I'll be left standing alone. For me, the value of that ball simply cannot be calculated.

Afterword

From the start, writing this book was fun and an amazing journey, one that changed the trajectory of my life. Putting words to paper is completely different from being a physician, and it became a wonderful diversion for me. I'm in awe of those who have mastered the skill of writing—an admiration that dates back to my days at Northwestern University, where I took a fair number of literature classes despite being a biology major. Faulkner was my favorite writer, or perhaps it was my professor who made the writer's world come to life for me. My daughter played a huge role in encouraging me to record the stories from my days on the court. I never intended to assemble these anecdotes into a book, yet three years later, that's exactly what happened. *Make Every Shot Count* ended up affecting me more than I could have imagined, and all in a good way.

The exercise of taking the time to organize my thoughts and record the experiences I perceived as most influential in my life brought about an intense understanding of how I became who I am. From childhood, basketball was my primary focus and dominated my very spirit. Yet despite my love for the game, I abruptly walked away, leaving those feelings behind to focus on academics in college. I knew that was what was needed to achieve my goal of becoming a doctor. Yet it took putting pen to paper to help me realize that I had repressed these experiences to the point where the stories were all but forgotten. As mentioned, it wasn't until many years later when I began to teach my daughter the fundamentals of the game that these memories bubbled up to the surface, and from there I wrote nonstop. I wrote late at night and when on call for the hospital. I wrote early in the morning before a twelve-hour work-day, and I wrote for eight hours every Saturday and

Sunday. Over the course of a full year, five hundred extremely disorganized pages came streaming out, and during this catharsis, I began to fully understand that I had written much more than stories. I was able to appreciate how basketball had prepared me for later success and taught me why I viewed the world as I did. It was an extraordinary exercise in self-awareness.

Fast-forward a few years when I started to wonder if I had missed my calling by going into medicine, since after all, basketball was the original plan. "I would've been a great coach," I boldly stated to my wife. "Maybe this medicine thing was not the right decision after all." Lisa pointed out that changing careers in my fifties wasn't a realistic option, but she encouraged me to reasonably pursue that dream. I took her advice and contacted some coaches I had become friendly with since moving to Virginia. Eight years later, it's been a tremendous ride.

My first reintroduction to the game was working at a summer camp for eight-to-sixteen-year-old kids. I told the coach I had befriended that I'd do anything just to be around the game again. I volunteered to set up cones, wash jerseys, put the balls back on the rack, and do anything else to help out. Despite my enthusiasm, it had been so long since I'd played that I wasn't sure I could still explain a simple bounce pass. I also wasn't confident that my skills were up-to-date. As I worked the camp and listened closely to the instruction in my less-than-cool, brand-new basketball shoes, I gained more experience and began to realize that the skills I had learned so many years before were not close to being outdated. In fact, they were needed now more than ever. With the encouragement of the coaches—now my valued friends—I've been an assistant at the varsity level for the past five years.

As a coach, my first love is practicing and teaching the fundamentals. Basic skills are so important, and that's where I feel I can contribute most. Although I'm very at home making split-second decisions in the operating room, I'm not quite ready for that mindset during a close contest on the court. I'm extremely thankful for the opportunity I have, knowing that I am exactly where I should be—working as both a coach and a physician. My sleep often suffers during the season, but I love being a part of two completely different worlds and feeling comfortable and capable in both.

My initial problem with *Make Every Shot Count* was that I wrote it without an audience in mind. The book has two very distinct sections, one about basketball and the other about medicine. Because I wasn't sure how these two parts were related, there was no way the reader could have been expected to make the connection. As the years passed, however, my perception of *Make Every Shot Count* has changed, and now I realize exactly how these two subjects fit together perfectly. I really like what the book is saying, and I'm proud of its message.

Make Every Shot Count is a book about both struggle and resilience. From the beginning of my basketball journey, I learned that I would never become an exceptional player without overcoming a multitude of obstacles. I pushed through adversity, stared down those who doubted me, and was never afraid to put in the time. I learned quickly that I was only as good as my last game and how essential it was to bounce back after a loss. I wasn't born with these abilities, but I was lucky to have had tremendous coaches and a support system that I was smart enough to listen to. Without integrating these values deeply, I could not have excelled in basketball. Without these traits being absorbed before the next phase of my life, I would have never had success in medicine. To become a doctor, you also are required to push through adversity, stare down those who doubt you, and not be afraid to put in the time. Every successful physician I know has incorporated these qualities. Of course, you can learn these skills from a multitude of sources; I just happened to have learned them on the court. It sounds cliché, but when you get knocked down, you have to be able to get up. You can't let a failure define who you are, or you can forget a career in medicine. It's far too stressful to be a physician, and you need this inner strength in addition to an incredible support system. The same goes for playing basketball, and in this case, the idea of being knocked down is often literal.

Make Every Shot Count simply is about learning resilience through a passion for the game of basketball, and then understanding the power this can provide to take you anywhere in life. That's the lesson, and it worked for me. This book also takes you to a place in time when young people were afforded independence and were allowed to learn from their own mistakes. The same can be said about the medical training I've described. Both worlds treated the learning process quite differently than they do today.

In this second edition of *Make Every Shot Count*, the thoughts and stories are the same as in the original publication, but the writing has been cleaned up. In addition to understanding the game of basketball at a higher level, I know that I have become a much better writer since the original manuscript was published in 2011. For that reason, I wanted to convey my message in a more appealing format.

I hope that you have enjoyed the book and these additional insights. Thank you so much for reading.

BR

Acknowledgments

First and foremost, I would like to thank my wife, Lisa. Without her wonderful skills and incredible support, this book would never have been possible. I would also like to thank my daughter, Ellen, who is the inspiration for this book and has been invaluable with her assistance every step of the way.

Thank you to Rob Clarick for getting through that early difficult draft and having the keen memory to make a difference. A special thanks to Craig Reeves for his review, encouragement, and "Craig-isms," which are always relevant and applicable. This same gratitude also goes out to Steve Kerr for his comments, support, and eloquent characterization of the often-overlooked true value of high school athletics.

A thank-you to John Haley, whose dedication and enthusiasm for basketball, especially at the high school level, is tremendous for the game. He was a terrific teammate on the floor and demonstrated that he retained those same attributes assisting me on this project. In addition, I want to thank Coach Bill Blindow for his encouragement and guidance. With incredible expertise, he taught us the game of basketball while emphasizing discipline, honesty, and respect—lessons that lasted long after the jump shot faded.

Of course, I have a great love and appreciation for the always-present support and opportunities afforded by my father, Philip A. Rosenfeld, MD, the quintessential physician and surgeon and a tremendous role model. This similarly goes to my mother, Roberta Rosenfeld, the "White Momma" to many of my friends, for providing a safe haven for those tougher times.

I would like to thank my editor, Christina Roth, for making this book readable and coherent with her incredible skills and professionalism.

ACKNOWLEDGMENTS

Finally, I am greatly indebted to all the coaches and role models I have had the privilege of knowing throughout my years on the court. We thought that we were learning and being taught basketball, but it was so much more than that. Finally, a huge thank-you to the orange ball. I am certain that my life would have been very different if our paths had not crossed.

About the Author

BRUCE ROSENFELD is a practicing urologist and a varsity basketball coach. His second book, *Unconscious Basketball*, is a companion to *Make Every Shot Count* and was written specifically to teach young middle school and high school athletes how to excel at the game while acquiring skills that will last a lifetime. This is the second edition of *Make Every Shot Count*.

CPSIA information can be obtained
at www.ICGtesting.com
Printed in the USA
LVHW012102051020
667983LV00007B/2069